PRAISE FOR *THE NERDY NURSE'S GUIDE TO TECHNOLOGY*

"Nurses are continuously adapting to the improvements in technology, often adding more time, hassle, and frustration to the clinical care process. But with Brittney Wilson's humor and tech-savvy tips, using EMRs, iPads, and smartphones makes patient care a lot more fun! The Nerdy Nurse's Guide to Technology *provides nurses with all the knowledge and tools they need to be successful in their nursing careers. This book is entertaining, informative, and full of personality! An absolute must-read!"*

–Donna Wilk Cardillo, MA, RN
The Career Guru for Nurses
"Dear Donna" columnist at *Nurse.com*
Expert blogger at *DoctorOz.com*

*"*The Nerdy Nurse's Guide to Technology *is invaluable for nurses struggling with the brave new world of health care IT. And if you don't know what that is–READ THIS BOOK. You'll be glad you did."*

–Theresa Brown, BSN, RN, OCN
Author of *Critical Care: A New Nurse Faces Death, Life, and Everything in Between*

"As a nerdy nurse myself, I have to say this book covers everything you need to know about smartphones, tablets, computers, apps, computer search engines, and basic software. It's beautifully written to help ANY nurse learn about and become comfortable with technology. (I learned a few things too!) We all know the use of technology is only going to expand to improve outcomes for our patients and make us better nurses."

–Kathy Quan, RN, BSN, PHN
Author, blogger (*TheNursingSiteBlog.com*), and QI nurse for hospice

"Written in a lively, engaging voice, Wilson's book brings technology to life and shows its relevance to every aspect of nursing. Her subject knowledge is extensive, and her enthusiasm for it is infectious. In Wilson's hands, nursing informatics is fun and fascinating, which is fortunate because the information in this book is absolutely essential to every nurse's practice. If this is what being a "nerdy" nurse is like, I want to be one, too."

–Tilda Shalof RN, BScN
Author of *A Nurse's Story, The Making of a Nurse* and
Opening My Heart: A Journey from Nurse to Patient and Back Again

"*The Nerdy Nurse's Guide to Technology is an exceptionally well written, comprehensive, and helpful resource on technology that nurses need and want to know about. Whether you are intimidated by computers, curious about social media, or fascinated by smartphones, this book will expand your knowledge—and you'll have fun reading it! I highly recommend it!*"

–Beth Boynton, RN, MS
Organizational Development Consultant and Author

"*Brittney Wilson has created an insightful primer on technology and nursing. The blend of practical applications with a conversational writing style engages the reader from the get-go! Nerdy Notes and Tech Tips get an A+ from this former professor and current clinical educator. This is a perfect fit for undergraduates studying basic concepts of nursing as well as the bedside nurse who lives and breathes technology each day.*"

–Lucy Megginson, PhD, RN
Director of Clinical Excellence, Floyd Medical Center

"*This book is a must-have for any nurse. There is no way to escape technology in our world today. Brittney Wilson does an incredible job of making it easy to understand how these tools can help any nurse! Whether you are looking for a place to start or tips for improving how you use your smartphone, this book has it covered.*"

–Robert Fraser, MN, RN
Registered Nurse, University Health Network
Order Set Developer, *PatientOrderSets.com*
Nurse, Author, and Digital Tool Strategist, *NurseRob.com*
Author, *The Nurse's Social Media Advantage*

"*Brittney Wilson brings to life the nerdy side of nursing from blogs, to social media, to electronic health records. All types of computer programs and applications that seem difficult are simplified into easily understandable language. After reading this book, all nurses will be able to express themselves through social media or their own incredible blogs. A pleasure to read!*"

–Epstein LaRue, RN, BS, CGM
Travel Nurse and author of the #1 Amazon eBook
Highway Hypodermics: Travel Nursing 2012

"*Brittney Wilson's book is packed with information that any nurse practicing today will appreciate. It's clear, readable, and fun.*"

–Carol Gino, RN, MA
Blogger and best-selling author of *The Nurse's Story* and other books
Publisher and CEO of aaha! Books, LLC

THE
NERDY NURSE'S
GUIDE TO
TECHNOLOGY

BRITTNEY WILSON, BSN, RN

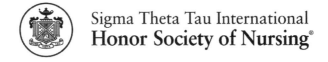

Sigma Theta Tau International
Honor Society of Nursing®

The Honor Society of Nursing, Sigma Theta Tau International (STTI), is a nonprofit organization whose mission is to support the learning, knowledge, and professional development of nurses committed to making a difference in health worldwide. Founded in 1922, STTI has 130,000 members in more than 85 countries. Members include practicing nurses, instructors, researchers, policymakers, entrepreneurs, and others. STTI's 486 chapters are located at 626 institutions of higher education throughout Australia, Botswana, Brazil, Canada, Colombia, Ghana, Hong Kong, Japan, Kenya, Malawi, Mexico, the Netherlands, Pakistan, Portugal, Singapore, South Africa, South Korea, Swaziland, Sweden, Taiwan, Tanzania, United Kingdom, United States, and Wales. More information about STTI can be found online at www.nursingsociety.org.

Sigma Theta Tau International
550 West North Street
Indianapolis, IN, USA 46202

To order additional books, buy in bulk, or order for corporate use, contact Nursing Knowledge International at 888.NKI.4YOU (888.654.4968/U.S. and Canada) or +1.317.634.8171 (outside U.S. and Canada).

To request a review copy for course adoption, email solutions@nursingknowledge.org or call 888.NKI.4YOU (888.654.4968/U.S. and Canada) or +1.317.634.8171 (outside U.S. and Canada).

To request author information, or for speaker or other media requests, contact Marketing, Honor Society of Nursing, Sigma Theta Tau International at 888.634.7575 (U.S. and Canada) or +1.317.634.8171 (outside U.S. and Canada).

ISBN: 9781937554385
EPUB ISBN: 9781937554392
PDF ISBN: 9781937554408
MOBI ISBN: 9781937554415

Library of Congress Cataloging-in-Publication data

Wilson, Brittney, 1985- author.
  The nerdy nurse's guide to technology / Brittney Wilson.
    p. ; cm.
  Includes bibliographical references.
  ISBN 978-1-937554-38-5 (book : alk. paper)—ISBN 978-1-937554-39-2 (ePub)—ISBN 978-1-937554-40-8 (PDF)—ISBN 978-1-937554-41-5 (MOBI)
  I. Sigma Theta Tau International, publisher. II. Title.
  [DNLM: 1. Nursing--trends. 2. Technology. 3. Electronic Health Records. 4. Internet. 5. Social Media. WY 16.1]
  RT50.5
  610.730285—dc23
                2013034948

First Printing, 2013

Publisher: Renee Wilmeth	**Principal Book Editor:** Carla Hall
Acquisitions Editor: Emily Hatch	**Development and Project Editor:** Emily Hatch
Editorial Coordinator: Paula Jeffers	**Copy Editor:** Heather Wilcox
Cover Designer: Michael Tanamachi	**Proofreader:** Andrew Kimmel
Interior Design/Page Layout: Rebecca Batchelor	**Indexer:** Jane Palmer

DEDICATION

To my late mother:

You taught me to read, even though you struggled with the words on the page yourself. Thank you for leading by example and preparing me to face life as a strong and passionate woman.

ACKNOWLEDGMENTS

So many people have contributed to this book in their own unique ways that it would probably take an entire book to acknowledge them properly. That being said, this section of the book is going to be relatively short and sweet, so if I forget to name you, please forgive me. You have my permission to pinch me (fairly hard) if you should have been included and you weren't.

I would like to thank Emily Hatch and the entire team at the Honor Society of Nursing, Sigma Theta Tau International. Your patience, persistence, and feedback were what motivated me to complete this work. Thank you for transforming me from a blogger to an author.

I would like to thank my fantastic boss, Keith Driskell, for taking a chance on me and allowing me to realize my nursing informatics dreams. I am so grateful that I get to work with a great boss like you who appreciates me for my strengths and helps me grow. A huge thank you to the home health nurses and staff who have accepted me with open arms and appreciate what I have to offer. I would also like to thank my clinical applications teammates for being able to handle my passion and nerdiness with charm to spare. Thank you, guys, for being loud, energetic, and talented. You make work fun! A special thanks to Carrie Hudgins for being my wingwoman and helping me out whenever I get in a bind.

I would like to give special thanks to my friends who have been very supportive and excited for me! Extra-special thanks go to Kate-Madonna Hindes. Even though we're halfway across the country from one another, you're always there for me and have helped me learn and grow as a person and as a social media personality.

To my nursing instructors and mentors: I appreciate your patience and your words of wisdom. You gave me strength to become a nurse and have no doubt passively influenced thousands of lives. Michelle Dorsett, your sense of humor and kindness really gave me strength at a difficult time in my nursing career. Stacy Ray, I miss you dearly and will always be thankful to have had the pleasure of working with you and learning from you.

Without a doubt, my readers at *The Nerdy Nurse* have played a large role in the creation of this book. Thank you for dealing with my subpar grammar, rambling, rants, and raves. You've helped me grow as a writer, and I hold you very dear to my heart.

To my family: You have all played a big role in my life and are a support system when I need it most. You are all very important to me, but I especially want to make sure that I recognize my aunts. I appreciate you all and feel that each one of you is like a little piece of my late mother.

Dad, we've had our ups and downs. I am so glad that you are in my life and are so supportive.

Mark, thank you for going along for the ride on whatever roller coaster my career takes me and for being supportive of me the whole way.

Ty, I am terribly sorry that I would not allow you to type gibberish on my manuscript. You've given me the joy of motherhood and have brought so much clarity to many of the things that my mother would say. I love you dearly, darling, and you have made me a much better person than I ever thought possible. You are why they invented the art of caring, and the world is a much better place because you are in it. I cannot wait to see what you accomplish with your life. Your contributions to this book are greater than you will ever realize, and I am so honored to be your mother.

Every experience in my life, good or bad, has molded me into the person I am today and has ultimately made this book possible. If you've been a part of any of it, thank you.

ABOUT THE AUTHOR

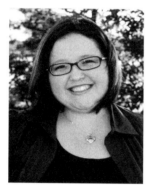

BRITTNEY WILSON, BSN, RN

Wilson is an informatics nurse with a passion to improve health care and everyday life through the use of technology. She identifies herself as a patient, nurse, and technology advocate and actively blogs on related topics at *TheNerdyNurse.com*.

She attended Georgia Highlands College in Rome, Georgia, where she obtained an associate of science in nursing. She later attended the University of West Georgia in Carrollton, Georgia, where she obtained a bachelor of science in nursing.

Wilson has worked with Johnson & Johnson on its Campaign for Nursing's Future. She is a national speaker and has given presentations for the international EMR provider Meditech. She also works as a brand ambassador for *Scrubs* magazine's popular nursing website and print publication.

When Wilson isn't brushing up on new technology to stay abreast of evolving digital changes, she enjoys spending time with her son, Ty, and her husband, Mark.

Her parents instilled in her a good work ethic and the knowledge that she could be anything she wanted. Even though her late mother was functionally illiterate, she ensured that Wilson always knew the importance of education and taught her as much as she could herself. Wilson's father instilled a love of technology in her from an early age and has always given her the benefit of allowing her to be her own nerdy, weird, outspoken, and opinionated self.

Her early years in nursing were made increasingly difficult by a year of many changes. Between 2008 and 2009, she became a nurse, got married, broke her leg, lost her mother, and had a baby. All the while, she was being bullied at work by other nurses.

Her struggles to overcome her experience with lateral violence and educate others on this issue led her to blogging and social media. She is active online in the nursing social media community, and her blog is consistently ranked as one of the top nursing blogs.

You can connect with her online by visiting her blog, *The Nerdy Nurse*; connecting with her on Twitter, @TheNerdyNurse; or finding her on Facebook, facebook.com/thenerdynurse.

TABLE OF CONTENTS

INTRODUCTION

"We live in a society exquisitely dependent on science and technology, in which hardly anyone knows anything about science and technology."

–Carl Sagan

There isn't a day that goes by during which you can escape technology. It powers our homes, propels our cars, grows our food, and provides our entertainment. Even if you do not consider yourself to be a technologically savvy person, chances are you use technologies every day that your great-grandmother could hardly even dream of.

If we are all constantly using technology, why are we sometimes so afraid of it? What is it about colorful graphics, brushed aluminum cases, and island-set keys that is so intimidating? Is the soft hum of a fan annoying? Is the smooth glass of a tablet off-putting? Are Chiclet-style keyboards pretentious? How can something as small and brilliant as a smartphone be of no interest to so many? Are you afraid that you will fail if you try to use it? Perhaps you are confident that it will be of no benefit to you and therefore you have no interest in learning to use technology—or maybe it's just a lack of free time.

I get having a lack of free time. In fact, I think almost all nurses get this lack of free time. We're busy at work, at home, and anywhere and everywhere in between. For most of us, there is hardly an extra moment to waste on learning something new if it isn't going to benefit us or enhance our nursing practice in any way.

Time is a treasure. So many of us have so little these days, and there isn't a single thing that can be done well without investing at least some measure of it. So feeling apprehensive about giving up any of your precious time on something that you are not sure is worthwhile is completely understandable. But what you should understand is that technology *is* worth the time and—here's the key point to all of this—it ultimately *can* and *will* save you time. Technology can improve your life in more ways than you can imagine, and it can connect you to the world on a global level. It can broaden your horizons and open your eyes to the world's culture, art, music, and literature. But ultimately, what you should gain from this book is the keen understanding that technology can help make you a better nurse.

Nursing is a career in which you should never be bored. Most nurses probably don't even remember what being bored feels like. There is always new information to learn, and changes are constantly taking place. Technology is one of those changes. The pages of this book include some examples of how technology can improve patient care and ultimately make you a better nurse.

I've encountered so many nurses who instantly put up a wall when discussions about using technology occur. "I'm not a computer person," they say, or "I don't know anything about computers." But these words are often coming from nurses who use computers for many hours of their nursing shifts. These nurses have good command of the basic skills needed to tackle any technology they choose, but for some reason, they don't seem to have confidence in their abilities to use technology well. They can navigate the hospital's electronic medical records (EMRs), print documents, and document their care without any difficulty—yet they claim they have no computer skills.

Nurses, why are you selling yourselves short? You are far more talented and capable than you ever give yourself credit for. You are masters of adaptation and can thrive in any environment you choose. You understand and embrace your adaptability when delivering patient care, but somehow you seem to forget these skills when it comes to embracing new technologies.

In my work as an informatics nurse, I meet many nurses and other health care team members who are absolutely terrified of breaking their computers. If any messages or dialogue boxes pop up on the screen, they automatically click "no" regardless of what the message says. Their instinct is to automatically decline whatever the computer is asking even though, more often than not, they haven't actually read the message. Their fear of viruses, spyware, and other computer baddies just takes hold of them, and they don't trust anything that pops up on their screen.

Before you click anything on your computer screen, you should read it! What if it told you that if you clicked "no," you would wipe out the entire Internet, and you just swiftly clicked anyway? You'd have hoards of nerds crying in the corner because they could no longer get online, all because you didn't bother to read the message on your computer screen.

Don't worry, it isn't possible for you to wipe out the entire Internet in one click, but it *is* possible to enable or disable functionality on your computer if you aren't paying attention. Before jumping to conclusions and hurriedly clicking on boxes to make them go away, make sure you read them. The people who design computer software are pretty good about giving you notifications about what's going on. If you're using a computer for work or for play, these messages are meant for you.

The reality is that computers are made to be so user-friendly that you really have to make a special effort to break them. Those messages and dialogue boxes that pop up on the screen or appear in a bar on your web browser are usually your computer's friendly little reminder that it wants to ask you a question. Closing the box without even reading it is not the correct response and may prevent you from accomplishing things you want to do.

Just remember, you are smarter than the computer. Don't let your fear of the unknown prevent you from getting what you want out of technology.

We have to stop treating technology as an invader within our little world of nursing care. We have to stop pretending that computers and mobile devices are somehow going to replace us at the bedside. They can make a million and one robots, electronic ICUs, and completely automated and reliable computerized decision support tools, but they still will not come close to replacing the value of one highly skilled and experienced nurse. And no computer can come close to capturing the essence of nursing: caring.

A growing number of nurses and other health care professionals are taking the time to see the value of technology in this field. They have left the bedside and are using their nursing skills to help patients in a different way by using clinical informatics. They are building and deploying EMR systems and other health care technologies. But they aren't just implementing EMRs because the government told them to; they are working to make sure that systems are user-friendly and ultimately have the patients' best interests at heart. These clinical professionals are working behind the scenes to help you deliver good patient care.

For informatics nurses to be successful, we rely on the support of others. By being eager to learn, you can help us help you deliver better patient care. And we should be able to help each other be less frustrated with our jobs!

Technology should be seen and used as an aide to delivering nursing care. If it is a barrier, then we need to break down those walls and make it useful for the care you give. Technology, like most things in life, becomes what you make of it. If you make it difficult and useless, then it will be difficult and useless. But if you make it prominent and valuable, then you might find that you not only experience increased satisfaction in your job performance but are a happier nurse overall.

Take the time to see past the difficulty of learning a new technology, and instead focus on the light at the end of the tunnel. If you have trouble seeing the light, then squint a little. See it yet? OK, just take my word for it—it's there. You will see that technology improves patient outcomes, decreases length of hospital stays, and decreases the cost of health care. And if you squint even harder, you might even see yourself enjoying the technology you use and perhaps even becoming a technology advocate yourself.

I have no doubt that you take excellent care of your patients. If you didn't, you wouldn't be taking the time to read this book. The very fact that you want to learn more about using technology in nursing proves that you have what it takes. A desire to learn and an opportunity to use what you have learned are the primary requirements of becoming a nurse who is skilled in the technologies needed to continue to provide excellent patient care in the years to come.

Take a deep breath, settle in for a while, and let *The Nerdy Nurse's Guide to Technology* help you get your toes wet in the magnificent ocean of innovation and wonder that is technology.

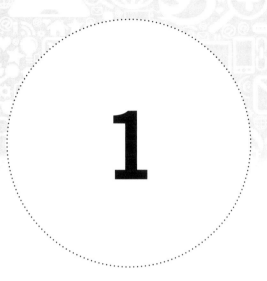

HAVE FUN WITH WHAT TECHNOLOGY HAS TO OFFER!

When you were in nursing school, you likely had to spend countless hours in the library, researching nursing issues, theorists, and other topics for your papers and care plans. You found your NANDAs (the acronym representing the North American Nursing Diagnosis Association, although nurses use this term to refer to nursing diagnosis) and drug information by tediously looking through pages of information to uncover a few relevant details. You painstakingly wrote your papers over and over, first by hand and then meticulously on a typewriter. If you were lucky, the model you used had a memory, and if you weren't, you were forced to trash hours of work just for misplacing a punctuation mark. To read a nursing journal, you actually had to have a subscription to the publication or access to a hard copy. You might spend

$20 to $30 just making copies of resources to write a single research paper. This process had to be repeated multiple times, costing you money you really didn't have to spend as a broke college student. But you toughed it out because you needed the information and had no other means to get it. In the end it was all worthwhile—here you sit, a licensed nurse.

Today's student nurses do not have to deal with nearly this amount of heartache when it comes to doing research. They seldom have to go to an actual library. They can even purchase their nursing textbooks in a digital format and avoid lugging around 50 pounds of books every semester. That's just unfair, right? Even though nursing school is still rigorous and difficult by any standards, some aspects are a breeze compared to what many had to face while earning their degrees. I'm not saying it's easy, because it's not. But I am saying that technology has really helped lessen some of the monotony of tasks. As much as a librarian or stern teacher will tell you that learning the Dewey Decimal System builds character, the fact is that this skill is really only needed by librarians.

Researching a topic and writing a paper are now as simple as making a few clicks on the mouse and spending a few hours in front of a computer screen. In nursing school, I could crank out a five-page, well-researched paper in a day—not because I'm that good, but because I knew how to use technology to my advantage. "So what?" you might be thinking. "I'm not in school. How does this relate to me?" Oh! I'm so glad you asked!

If you know how to use technology to find information, there are practically no limitations to what you can learn. Whether you're interested in getting a nursing certification, pressure-washing your house, or learning the side effects of Zoloft, it's all available to you. No more thumbing through books and stray bits and pieces of information that may be helpful. You can now find countless numbers of videos, articles, and images to address any need you have.

It is now easier than ever to learn. Whether you are interested in learning about improving patient outcomes using evidence-based practices in nursing care or learning how to build a website, technology can quickly and easily provide the answers. Plus, accessing it is a whole lot of fun!

It's really quite mind-blowing to think of all the innovations we've made in technology in the past 20 years. It may seem as though everyone is connected on Facebook and attached to their mobile devices, but the unfortunate reality is that everyone *isn't* connected. I meet nurses every day who claim to have no interest in learning about new technologies and put up walls when I speak passionately about all the great things you can do with them. Sometimes these nurses look at me like I'm stark naked running up and down Broad Street when I passionately speak about all the things technology can do for them. They don't get it, and I understand. We all have our passions, and being nerdy isn't for everyone, but it certainly can be for nurses.

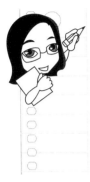

NERDY NOTE

Let's just clear something up here: Nerd is not a four-letter word—well, technically it is, but you get the point. Being called nerdy is a compliment! It means you have the ability to grasp concepts in emerging technology and understand how computers can improve your life and the lives of the patients you care for.

I wear my nerd stamp like a badge of honor because it makes it possible for me to positively affect lives of far more patients.

The world is so different these days. Technology changes every day, and we are advancing so rapidly that it can be really hard to keep up. For some, accepting these changes can be even harder. Even the nerdiest of nerds, myself included, can have their minds blown from time to time. Sometimes it's even hard to fathom and comprehend what I've seen in my short lifetime. There are moments when even the best of us find ourselves completely overwhelmed. And there is nothing at all wrong with this. Even though it seems that others just "get it," the real truth is that everyone struggles with technology on some level, even if they are too proud to admit it. I want you to know that it's OK to feel like a fish out of water. It's OK to be confused and overwhelmed sometimes. But it's not OK to quietly let others completely surpass you in their technology skills. You owe it to yourself and to your patients to be informed.

The technology we have today is worlds away from what many thought we might have 30 years ago. When you were a kid, if someone had walked up to you and said that by the time you were an adult, a revolutionary device that contained all the world's knowledge could fit in your pocket, there's no doubt that you would have been skeptical. But the fact is that technology has given us greater access to information that we've ever had before. Even with all this power and information, many of us merely use this technology to write on walls and look at funny pictures of cats. Perhaps ancient Egyptians were way ahead of their time with their hieroglyphics and cat-worshipping habits!

As a nurse, you can access any information you may need to help you educate a patient or perform a procedure (except experience, of course—only time can give you that!). But if you're a new nurse or you want to brush up on the latest information about the newest procedure or the most recent and best published practices, technology is where it's at.

NERDY NOTE
Egypt—wait, what?

Facebook is all about writing on walls. It's like modern-day hieroglyphics (and people's posts are just as permanent).

Today, entire online communities are devoted to sharing cute and funny cat pictures. There are thousands upon thousands of them. I don't completely understand the allure of these cat pictures, but even I've found myself consumed by them at various points. If you have a few hours to spare, check out http://icanhas.cheezburger.com and www.lolcats.com, but don't say I didn't warn you.

As nurses, we all had to carry our share of thick textbooks through college. Ebook technology is now available at a fraction of the cost, and with readers widely available at affordable rates, carrying an entire library of heavy textbooks is no longer necessary. A smartphone or a tablet provides access to all this information in a compact format, allowing you to carry it wherever you go. One of these tools will give you easy access to relevant drug data, information about a patient diagnosis, or acceptable ranges for lab values. You can get all this information from downloading mobile apps, searching through ebooks, or surfing the Web.

Here are just a few examples of information you can find using technology:

+ Aftercare standards for a hysterectomy

+ Normal HGB for a pediatric patient

+ Instructions to perform a Foley catheterization using aseptic technique

+ Proper procedure for staple removal

+ Possible side effects and contraindications for medications

These examples are merely scratching the surface of the type of information that technology can give you, but I think you get the idea.

WHY YOU SHOULD WANT MORE TOOLS IN YOUR HANDY-DANDY TOOLBOX

The more tools you have in your nursing toolbox, the better you can take care of your patients. Information and the means to get more information are valuable tools. However, many nurses believe that they already learned all they need to know when they were in nursing school or through their experience in the field. But any good nurse knows that the moment you stop learning is the moment you become dangerous. You should always add to your informational toolbox. Practices and standards change over time, and you have to be ready to adapt.

You've likely heard that you need to be using technology. If you are reading this book, then you probably even have an interest in doing so. You might have reasons for wanting to become more comfortable with technology, or you might still be on the edge of determining whether doing so is worth your time and energy. To be quite honest, most people probably couldn't give you a clear-cut answer to the question "Why should I be embracing technology?" And they certainly couldn't tell you the answer to the question "How can using technology make me a better nurse?"

The reality is that it's difficult for most people to tell you why you should be using technology and be interested in learning more about it. The lovers of technology—nerds and geeks and the like—just get it. We know what it does for us, and we know that the experience is different for everyone. Ultimately, it's up to you to determine how far into the nerd forest you wish to venture, but I'd probably recommend you stop somewhere before LARPING. Anywhere before that is golden, and you'll be happy with your newfound digital savvy.

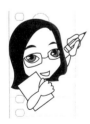

NERDY NOTE

LARPING = Live Action Role Playing. It's mostly adults who like to pretend they are video game characters. If it sounds weird to you, that's because it is.

I go pretty deep into the nerd forest, but I draw the line at LARPING.

I can tell you are a smart person who is no doubt ready and willing to learn. How, you say? Well you're reading this book, aren't you?

To reward your attention and to show appreciation for your willingness to learn something new, I'm going to explain exactly how technology can make you a better nurse and assist you in providing excellent patient care. I'll even make sure you learn a few tips and tricks to make using technology a more enjoyable experience overall.

A DESIRE TO IMPROVE YOUR NURSING CARE

The second you get your nursing license, you are considered responsible and knowledgeable enough to take care of patients. Depending on your employer's policy, you may be assigned your very own patients with minimal supervision in a matter of weeks. You now have lives in your hands and are responsible for the care of a sick and aging population of adults and maybe even children.

Even if you read every chapter, studied every note, and aced every test, the knowledge that you gained in nursing school is somewhat finite. New information is always being discovered, and standards in patient care are always improving. As long as evidence exists, there will always be ways to improve your care that stem from evidence-based practices.

You might argue that you can continue your education via hospital in-services, print nursing journal subscriptions, or courses at a local college, but you'd be drastically limiting yourself. This approach makes the process of expanding your nursing knowledge rigid and out of your control. If you want to be the best nurse possible, you owe it to yourself and your patients to expand your nursing knowledge in other ways.

If you are a nurse who works in a hospital, you likely already know that many hospital administrators offer in-services that are conducted by device sales personnel. They are only interested in ensuring that you know how to properly use their products. They are not up to date on all the research related to a particular procedure and are really only there to sing the praises of their devices and the manufacturers or vendors that employ them. Their short demos don't usually give you contact hours, which are needed for continuing education (CE) requirements, upon completion and are usually a shortcut for hospital management to check off a few boxes to meet regulations and guidelines. Many of them provide you with little information regarding ways to improve nursing care, other than being able to use a specific new piece of equipment that the hospital management likely bought primarily based on price.

If you are lucky, you might be among the privileged few who have excellent nursing education opportunities at their hospitals, but these chances are happening less often these days due to cuts in Medicare and other health care budget concerns. If you are lucky enough to have a team of nursing educators on staff, then you might have courses offered frequently on a variety of topics. However, the classes may or may not be offered at times that are convenient to you, and they may or may not discuss topics that you find interesting or relevant.

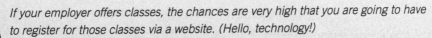

CODE CAUTION

If your employer offers classes, the chances are very high that you are going to have to register for those classes via a website. (Hello, technology!)

Your employer likely has an intranet (in-facility network) that you will navigate to the registration page. Depending on your setup, your login details may already be saved on your employer's computer. If they are not and you must log in to a computer generically, you will need to identify yourself when you register. This may be in the form of your employee number, or you may be asked to create a unique user name and password. I know, it's a pain. But you need to make sure that you are registering for a class and not accidentally registering someone else. If you have to create a user name and password, make sure that you can remember them because you may need to use them again to access the class. If you are worried about remembering passwords and user names, several password management apps are available for your smartphone that can help you keep things straight.

SO YOU WANT TO BE A BIG SHOT: IS HIGHER EDUCATION RIGHT FOR YOU?

You may decide that you want to further your nursing education in a more substantial way. To do this, you can go back to school to pursue an advanced degree, likely a BSN, MSN, or PhD. If you are taking this big step in your nursing career, I applaud you.

But I've talked to so many nurses who have absolutely no desire to go back to school. They've earned an LPN, ADN RN, or even BSN and are convinced that their current degrees are as far as they need to go. They remember all the trials and tribulations of going to nursing school and do not want to go through the same agonies again. They think that they are either too old or too tired to put up with the drama. You may very well feel this way yourself.

Many options aside from the traditional nursing school setting will allow you to earn a higher degree in nursing. There are programs that are totally online, combination courses, and courses that are based primarily in the classroom. However, most programs require at least some interaction with the Internet and new technologies. Being uncomfortable with technology will put you at a disadvantage.

However, some people like to dive right into the deep end of the pool. Taking online classes may just be the motivator you need to break out of your technophobic shell. In addition to helping you improve your technology skills, online learning can be a great method to fit higher education into your schedule, because you can usually complete assignments and attend lectures on your own time. Many find that with the added personal freedom of online courses, there is less stress involved, and they have a much more enjoyable school experience.

It would be nearly impossible to manage the assignments, lecture notes, course work, communication, and schedules of nursing students without the aid of computers. As we discussed earlier, writing a research paper alone is a painful task without the use of a modern word-processing program and the Internet. If it is important to you to get a higher degree, then you are going to have to face the facts and get on board with technology. Who knows—you may just be a budding nerd waiting to bloom!

Multiple studies and research support the benefits of higher education in the nursing population. In an article published in the *Journal of the American Medical Association*, Aiken, Clarke, Cheung, Sloane, and Silber (2003) confirm that an increase in nursing education levels leads to a decrease in patient mortality rates: "In hospitals with higher proportions of nurses educated at the baccalaureate level or higher, surgical patients experienced lower mortality and failure-to-rescue rates." This by no means is meant as an insult to any nurse who is not at this level of education, but it's a clear argument for higher education in nursing. I am an advocate of continuing education. It's not a black and white situation, but higher education can help you save more lives, and if saving a life isn't a good-enough argument, I am not sure what would be.

ESTABLISH YOURSELF AS AN ASSET TO YOUR EMPLOYER

Being able to learn new technologies quickly can prove extremely valuable in a nurses station. The regulations and requirements for nursing and patient care are constantly changing, as does the related technology. It seems like hospital administrators everywhere are implementing or changing their electronic medical records (EMR) systems to keep up with the times and be in compliance with government-driven programs, such as Meaningful Use.

Even if you haven't heard the term "Meaningful Use," there is no doubt that you are experiencing the side effects of its implementation. Health care organizations have to comply with these government guidelines to get monetary compensation initially and then to continue getting Medicare reimbursement after that. We'll go over Meaningful Use in greater detail in Chapter 7, but for now you should know that it involves collecting data in a methodical way by using EMRs to improve patient care.

BECOME A SUPER USER

If you are a nurse who can quickly learn a system and train others, then you may be referred to as a Super User. Being a Super User shows that you have the ability to train others on new technology. You are a go-to person when others have difficulty using EMRs, whether it means implementing a new intervention or remembering how to access a seldom-used assessment. You may be invited to additional training that may take place onsite or off. If you are a nurse who likes taking on new challenges and sharing your knowledge with others, this is an area where you can shine.

Some organizations have a formal process for selecting Super Users, and they even receive additional pay for taking on this role. Other organizations are less formalized and encourage anyone to step up to the plate and rise to the challenge. You should speak with your manager about your employer's Super User process to learn how you can become a part of the team.

TECH TIP

An excellent way to improve your computer skills and gain confidence in documenting on an EMR is to volunteer to be a Super User. If your employer is going through a software implementation, this is an excellent time to offer your services. If you are already using an EMR system, then you can contact your manager to express your interest in becoming a Super User.

This initiative will cement your dedication to better learning EMR technology and wanting to be a resource to others. This is also a great skill to list on a resume, so if you have an opportunity to become a Super User, take it. If there isn't already an opportunity, make one. It usually requires only a little additional work and yields many benefits.

If your organization does not have designated Super Users and you're ready for a challenge, you should suggest that this process be implemented. This is an excellent tool for leadership to emerge and take control in difficult times of change. These nurses are seen as resources and often get recognized for their contributions to the team. Keep in mind that these responsibilities should not be restricted to charge nurses and managers alone; there needs to be at least one Super User on each shift.

Being a Super User is an excellent line item to add to a resume. You can list any of the skills you learned and accomplishments you made doing this role. Potential employers are really interested in nurses who like to take on challenges and educate others.

One of the best reasons to become a Super User is that doing so will make you an asset to your employer and your coworkers. You can provide leadership and guidance to others who struggle with change. You can help ensure that patients are getting the best care possible by making sure that nurses know the EMR system fluidly. This will also help you gain an increased level of confidence with new computerized equipment. Getting acquainted with new technologies is important because you need to be able to use them and educate your patients about them.

UTILIZE COMPUTER-BASED EQUIPMENT AND PROGRAMS ON THE JOB

Without even considering EMRs, there are so many ways that nurses use technology to deliver patient care, such as computerized IV pumps, computer-based medication dispensers (these go by many names, including AccuDose and Pyxis), supply rooms with computerized inventory and charge processes, and computer-driven scheduling for nurses and other health care team members. There are even computer-driven billboards advertising emergency department (ED) wait times and apps that let ED patients check in online.

If you learn how to operate the computerized IV pump, you can train other nurses on how to properly use it. You can find out the best method to ensure patient safety and fluidity in your process. If you are timid about using a computerized pump to deliver infusions, you may make a mistake that could cost a patient's life. Patients and family members are often keenly aware of nurses who are uncomfortable using a new technology, so they may be extracritical of your performance if you appear uneasy about using equipment.

IV pumps can be more than just computerized; they can be smart! Many pumps have the ability to scan in IV medications directly on the pumps themselves, verify against the patient's current medication administration record (MAR), and automatically set for the correct time and medication dosage. They can wirelessly transmit this data back to the EMR system and document the type and amount of medication delivered. Advances like these decrease the possibility of inaccurately setting up a pump. For instance, as you likely already know, many medications must be delivered over long periods of time to prevent phlebitis when using antibiotics that are vesicants. The pumps can help you determine whether you are delivering the medication at a safe and effective rate without the need to consult another source. A prime example of how this can be helpful is in ensuring you are selecting the proper flow for such medications as potassium, which can cause death or cardiac anomaly when administered inappropriately.

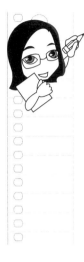

NERDY NOTE

Be sure to check with your manager or charge nurse to determine which type of pumps you have in your department and which capabilities they have. If smart pumps are available on the floor, make sure that you are trained on how to use them properly. They may have many features that will increase safety for your patients, including patient scanning and dose calculation. If you have electronic pumps that are not smart, make sure that you are calculating and inputting your medications correctly.

You should always remember that you are the nurse and are responsible for caring for your patient. Smart pumps and other technological advances can help you deliver patient care, but they are no replacements for good clinical judgment.

Computer-based medication dispensers can be useful in preventing you from delivering the wrong medication to a patient. Depending on the model of your machine, it may be able to limit the items you get out of the system. Narcotics, for example, are usually locked in an individual drawer and require you to enter the count remaining when you remove a dose from the system. This is an additional safeguard to the multiple checks that go into place prior to a patient getting a medication. It also gives a definitive record of when you pulled medication for a patient. Computer-based medication dispensers can be used for auditing and ensuring that patients are getting the medications their nurses are charging to their accounts.

Supply rooms with computerized inventory processes help hospitals with cost-saving measures. Instead of charging patients a standard fee for supplies and equipment, computerized inventories can ensure that patients are only being charged for what they are actually receiving. These systems also help to ensure that stock levels of supplies stay in check. Any nurse who has worked the floor knows that few situations are more annoying than having to go to another floor to get supplies for a procedure (especially when an irritated physician is waiting at the bedside).

Computerized inventory systems can be linked through a hospital and manage the overall inventory of supplies that are on hand. Some sophisticated software programs can even notify you when supplies are running low. These systems help ensure that patients are only charged for items that are needed for their care, but it is vital to use them properly to ensure that your unit is stocked with the supplies you need.

As a nurse, you will need to be aware of how to manage a computerized inventory system at the basic level. Doing so will likely require you to select a patient from a list and then scan the items that you will need for that patient. It is important to know how to use this system so that you can do it quickly and accurately. If you repeatedly use an item without scanning it out, then the inventory system will not accurately reflect the amount available, and you may find yourself out of a supply for a procedure when you really need it. If you think scanning items is inconvenient, try running to another floor to find ostomy supplies when your patient's bag has just exploded.

GO ON—STEP UP TO THAT PLATE!

You can also use technology to advance your career in other ways. You may decide to head up a project providing clinician education in the form of an in-service. You can easily research your chosen topic on the Internet and use such editing software as Microsoft Word or Publisher to create a brochure. You can use a high-end printer to print crisp images for a visual aid. You can even get a little crafty and use a digital paper cutter to cut out letters and other shapes for eye-popping posters.

Educational sessions and in-services always need to be cleared with management. They may want to review your educational materials to ensure that they comply with policies and procedures that are already in place. They may also want you to give the demonstration to additional groups of people.

If you are thinking of offering an educational in-service, your first step should be to ask your manager which guidelines you need to follow. At this point, you will only need to have an idea of your topic and your audience. If management accepts the pitch, then you will need to do your research and create your printed materials. You should provide this information to management for review prior to scheduling the in-service. After everything has been approved, you can schedule the in-service and make sure you are ready to give your presentation.

If you are presenting for nurses to get state-approved CEs, you will need to do additional research on what your state requires. This might be as simple as a written test or survey after an educational session, but it is better to check before you do all the work.

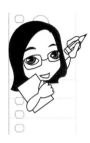

NERDY NOTE

Microsoft Word or Google Docs will meet many of your needs for document creation, whether it be a brochure, poster, or flyer. These word-processing programs can handle most text and graphic demands you throw at them. Many great tutorials and templates are available online if a feature in one of the programs intimidates you.

You can use technology to take the initiative on projects and showcase your leadership skills by organizing an online fund-raiser for a worthy cause. If you are hosting an event with many participants, an online sign-up process can simplify some of your efforts. Of course, the computer won't be able to do everything for you, but it will certainly lend a helping hand. By organizing a fund-raiser, you'll not only impress your employer but also make a difference in the world.

If you are organizing an event and are looking for volunteers or contributors, a tool as simple as Google Forms can make your life a breeze. You can specify a series of questions and make the form as short or as long as you need. After people click on the link to the form, they are directed to a page where they will complete the information required. It will then appear in a neat spreadsheet alongside other responses received. This is just one of the many ways that technology can help you organize and make a greater impact on nursing and patient care.

TECH TIP

When it comes to learning how to effectively use technology, Google is your best friend. Many tutorials are available in article and video formats that will teach you how to do just about anything. If you ever find yourself confused or frustrated, just enter what you are trying to do into Google's search bar. You'll be pleasantly surprised at how many resources you will find on just about anything you need.

You can create a website or blog to give attention to a worthy cause or an area in which the public needs education. You can focus on nursing, public health, or community resources. You might create a website to showcase some of the great things that your hospital staff is doing in the community. Your facility is no doubt doing a lot for the patients and community it serves, so it deserves credit where credit is due.

You can go about creating a website or blog in many different ways. Google offers website templates as well as blogs that are free and easy to use. If you want to create a static piece of web real estate that will require little in the way of updates, then you should build a website. If you are looking to create something that can easily be updated, then design something built on a blog database. You can create free blogs by going to various websites, including www.blogspot.com or www.wordpress.com. We'll talk a little more about blogging and social media in later chapters.

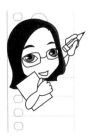

NERDY NOTE

Any activities involving your employer should be approved in advance. Any time your employer can be deduced or is already known, you should be sure to disclose that your opinions are your own and are not reflective of those of your employer.

BE A RESOURCE NERD TO OTHER NURSES AND STAFF

You don't always have be designated in any official way to educate other nurses. Even if your hospital does not have a Super User program, you can still take the time to show others tips and tricks. You can also educate others on the latest smartphone technology, digital cameras, cool websites, or maybe even the latest tablet. Pretty soon you'll be seen as the go-to person for tech questions. It's an awesome feeling to know that others are interested in your opinion and trust your advice.

You need to get on board with technology, because health care certainly is. Increased access to and forms of technology are affecting nearly everything and even helping patients decide whether to visit your ED. If you haven't already seen billboards advertising ED wait times, then you likely will soon. They proudly boast their wait times in the hopes that you will come visit their EDs. Although this type of advertisement is likely not every ED nurse's dream, it is a useful tool for patients who are deciding which ED they want to go to. If they don't happen to have the sign in view, then they can just log in to a smartphone app to check ED wait times.

If that isn't wild enough, some EDs even allow their incoming patients to preregister for ED visits online. Although many nurses believe that an ED visit should be reserved for those occasions where a patient is truly in need of critical care, many patients do appreciate and use this functionality.

It's not your job to agree with all the ways technology is used to improve health care, but it is your job to understand them and to be able to educate others. At the very least, you need to be able to inform your patients of any changes they might see in their care or methods that can increase their access to care.

Even if you only want to learn to appreciate technology outside the hospital setting, you will be able to pick up on new technologies at work more quickly than others. You will develop a "digital edge" that will make embracing change significantly easier while allowing you to be an asset to your coworkers and the health care organization that employs you.

The good news is that you can start small and build on your knowledge every day. You don't think that I started out being this nerdy, do you? But don't worry, picking up little tech skills will not make you a total nerd—it will simply prepare you to better handle the challenges that your chosen profession is going to throw at you.

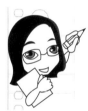

NERDY NOTE
I personally think that nerdiness is very appealing and suggest that you try it sometime. Then again, I'm a nerd.

YOUR PATIENTS WILL BENEFIT FROM YOUR NEWLY ACQUIRED TECH SAVVY

Many of your patients are already well acquainted with technology, but it is likely that a large portion, especially in the older population, is not. As a nurse, you can take opportunities to educate them about health information that can be found online. You can also discuss new devices, such as tablets, smartphones, and touch-screen computers. Your patients might also be interested in new innovations in diagnostic testing and procedures that can help them better identify and manage their illnesses.

Although your patients may often passively be exposed to others using technology, they may not fully understand the reasons for it. If you use bedside medication verification for patient care, many of your patients might be confused about why you always need to look at the computer or scan their bracelets. If you understand what technology is doing for you, then you can educate patients on the increased safety level that bedside medication verification provides. You can also let patients know that the computer has the most up-to-date information about their labs and medications. You need to electronically document the care you performed while it is still fresh in your mind so that it will be accurate in their medical records.

If you are able to tell your patients accurately and confidently why you are using the computer, your patients will have a new level of respect for your knowledge and expertise. You will not only provide excellent patient care but also provide tech-savvy education to meet your patients' needs. Sometimes a few extra minutes of explanation can really ease patients' minds and reduce their climbing stress levels.

I mentioned earlier some of the many innovations that are computer-based, excluding the EMR. Your patients many encounter many of these with increasing frequency as time progresses. You can help prepare them for the changes that technology will make in their health care experience by educating them.

EASY ACCESS TO THE FACTS YOU LEARNED IN NURSING SCHOOL

Earlier I mentioned some of the ways that technology can be used to obtain information, but what it all boils down to is that most people aren't capable of retaining everything they've ever known at any given time. Even the best nursing student didn't read every chapter of every textbook. If you combine this older, possibly forgotten information with the new information that is constantly being added to curricula and nursing practice, it's easy to see why all nurses need access to facts and figures that can help them provide better care.

We can all think of a time when we had a patient with one of those rare conditions that we seldom see. Instead of fumbling through a medical dictionary, you can easily go online and find accurate information about the condition. Most hospital administrators subscribe to educational resources that are vetted and contain evidence-based practices.

You likely are a pro at the many nursing procedures that you perform on a daily basis. Anything from medication reconciliation to IV insertion may be a breeze to you, but what if there is a better way? What if you could reduce the discomfort your patients experience and the length of time it takes you to perform the procedures? Are these techniques worth learning? It's worth taking the time to refresh yourself to make sure you are following procedures, if for no other reason than to confirm that you're an awesome nurse. Ultimately, you should want to know whether there have been any improvements in practice. You deserve to be the best nurse you can be.

A TOOL FOR PATIENT EDUCATION

Although you may know the basic information to tell patients about specific procedures or conditions, it is best to send them home with printed material. It is also helpful for them to know where they can find additional information. Your hospital management may subscribe to a resource that provides patient education via its website, or they may link to other websites with reputable information.

Most hospital administrators subscribe to education resources that will provide patients with the exact information they need, which can be printed and given to the patient upon discharge. You might recognize such names as Krames On-Demand, ExitCare, or perhaps EBSCOhost. These sources all provide patient educational materials that can be printed during your patients' stay or prior to their discharge. This information can be provided to reinforce instructions and education you've already given to patients while they were in the hospital. This additional information can help improve patient outcomes and leave a lasting impression on the patients.

The information found in these resources is vetted and evidence-based for your patients. Oftentimes these sites also provide patients with ways to access additional information. For example, patient education on diabetes might reference the American Diabetes Association website or a smartphone app to help diabetics keep track of their blood glucose levels.

These educational resources offer evidence-based practice guidelines and patient education printouts that are updated routinely and feature the most relevant and up-to-date information on patient conditions. Many hospital administrators attempt to make their own patient educational materials, which can be disjointed and may lack new information. If stacks of printouts are lying around, then patients may receive information about their conditions that is outdated and no longer relevant. The likelihood of this situation increases when this information is produced by hospital staff.

Some regulations require that the patient's education be specifically documented. If you give a patient a hospital-made patient education sheet, you need to also ensure that a copy of this sheet can be archived in the patient's medical record. Many times online systems keep logs of archived information, but sometimes they do not. When in doubt, you should always retain a copy and ask your manager which archival system exists for patient education and how you should be documenting the information given to the patient. As we all know, "If you didn't document, it wasn't done."

TECH TIP

Be sure to check your policies to determine which resources your hospital management deems appropriate for printed patient education. WebMD is usually *not* OK.

Although many patients may use WebMD in an effort to diagnosis themselves, its information may not be the most current available and may not be explicitly relevant to the patient. If your patients inform you that they are frequently visiting WebMD, you should use it as an educational opportunity to warn them of its potentially inaccurate information, increased unnecessary stress, and possible conflicts with what is appropriate for their plan of care. In short, it's OK for them to check out, but they should not see it as a holy grail of medical knowledge.

Also, if you are giving out educational materials to the patient, certain requirements must be met to maintain compliance standards. One of these includes making sure that a record of education that the patient was given is kept in the patient's medical record. If your hospital administrators aren't doing this, they will likely start soon!

EVIDENCE-BASED PRACTICE

If you want to deliver the best patient care possible, you want to employ evidence-based practices. It's been my experience that some nurses roll their eyes and thumb their noses at the sound of those words, but evidence-based practice is one of the greatest tools available in the pursuit of excellence in patient care. As nurses, we use evidence-based practice every day and often when we don't even realize it. Evidence-based practice is simply doing what works best through trial and error. When you started as a nurse, your technique wasn't nearly as good as it is now. You used the evidence you gained when you saw which methods and techniques worked best when you performed skills. Formal evidence-based practice is basically the same idea—trying to find the best methods to give patients the best care—except a ton of documentation and formal paperwork backs it up.

As time passes and technology progresses, evidence-based practice changes. The best method for doing a procedure today may not be the best a year from now. You can probably think of many practices that have changed since you became a nurse. If you're not learning these new methods, then you are doing the patient a disservice. When was the last time you put Betadine in a Foley catheter bag or used an actual needle to inject medications into a patient's IV line? The reason this is no longer done is because many experiments were performed to determine whether this actually improved patient outcomes or may even have been a potential safety risk. In the Betadine example, there was no significant impact, so this practice was stopped.

You can use technology to access the information that helps form these guidelines and best practices. If you're like many other nurses, you need to know more than just "do this"; you need to know *why* you are going to "do this." You need to know the benefits and the risks. You need to know the background. If you want this information, you will likely have to find it yourself, and there is no better place to start than Google and the Internet.

WAYS TO OBTAIN INFORMATION

With advances in technology, all the information in the world can be carried around with you in an object that is roughly the size of a magazine (or a cassette tape, if you're using a smartphone!). Even though tablets are becoming more affordable and more commonplace, they are not the only way to access information—smartphones and desktop computers also play a large role. The key is having a connection to the Internet, preferably via a broadband connection. With a broadband connection, you will be able to enjoy your technology with much more speed and without the burden of wires.

Countless devices make connecting to the Internet almost effortless. Whether it's a tablet, smartphone, laptop, desktop, Mac, or PC, you can easily get online via a home-based broadband solution or a mobile solution, such as a portable hotspot. Smartphones require data plans so that you can access the Web on the go, and most well-populated areas have access to near-broadband speeds. Many tablets have integrated broadband technology that allows you to access the Web anywhere with cell reception. As with smartphones, the speeds on these devices are near-broadband quality.

The main thing is to be connected and willing to learn. After that, everything else will fall into place.

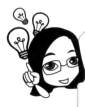

TECH TIP

A broadband connection is a type of high-speed Internet access that can be delivered in various forms. You might also commonly hear it referred to as cable, DSL, Wi-Fi, or just Internet. Unless you are plugging into a phone line and dialing up every time you want to connect to the Internet, you are probably using broadband.

Some major cities have broadband Internet connections that are completely wireless and operate on cell phone technology. This is a really new and innovative way to connect to the Internet that allows you to have a fast connection whether you are at home or around town for the same price. If you have access to Clear or another provider, you should totally check it out.

Something you should know is that not all broadband is created equal. For example, cable Internet is faster than DSL, and fiber optic (like Verizon FiOS) can even be faster than cable. So if you have family members who love their mobile devices, computers, and streaming media boxes, you need to make sure that you have enough Internet availability to meet their needs. For my connected family, DSL just doesn't cut it.

A hospital is going to have a high-speed internal network (intranet) and a broadband connection to the Internet. Depending on how your security is structured, you may or may not have access to the Internet at work.

TYING IT ALL TOGETHER

We've gone through the reasons why it's important to use technology and have started digging into the hows. Is your confidence level improving? If not, don't worry—we've still got lots to cover on many topics.

It's important to know that you're not going to be able to read a single book (even if it is as awesome as this one and written by The Nerdy Nurse herself) and find out all you need to know about using technology as a nurse. But you should gain a better grasp of how using technology can benefit you and pick up a few tips and tricks along the way.

I want you to take a moment to write down a few things:

1. Your fears related to using technology

2. Questions you would ask a tech guru if you had the chance

3. Tasks you would like to be able to do using technology

Did you write the answers down? It's important that you do. You can always pretend you did and keep reading, but the only way to ensure that you're honest about your answers now and later will be to put pen to paper (or fingers to keyboard, if you're feeling adventurous already!).

REFERENCE

Aiken, L.H., Clarke, S.P., Cheung, R.B., Sloane, D.M., & Silber, J.H. (2003, September 24). Educational levels of hospital nurses and surgical patient mortality. *Journal of the American Medical Association, 290*(12), 1617–1623. Retrieved from http://jama.jamanetwork.com/article.aspx?articleid=197345

2

THE INTERNET AND GOOGLE'S BRILLIANCE

The Internet is constantly changing and growing, and its content is highly dynamic and generated by its users. There are websites run by government agencies, small businesses, big businesses, political activists, teenage girls, middle-age men, nerdy nurses, and anyone and everyone in between. Because the content is created by people, there is always a chance that it may be wrong. However, if you stick with resources created by people who are authorities on their topics, you can pretty much bet that the information provided is accurate.

TECH TIP

As the saying goes, don't believe everything you read on the Internet. More than likely, a majority of what you read on the Internet has been skewed or manipulated in some way. You should know that many blogs and websites are written by individuals who may not have any real authority or expertise on the topics they are writing about. It's up to you to play detective to determine whether a site has merit.

You should check out the credentials of the authors and confirm that they know about the subjects they are writing about. If the content does not list an author, that may be a red flag, unless, of course, it comes from a trusted organization.

In short, don't let the Internet make you believe that gullible is not in the dictionary.

From ways to tile a bathroom floor to journal references for writing assignments, somebody, somewhere, has written about just about every topic you could think of on the Internet. More than just a repository for information, the Internet allows us to be better resources for our employers and to make connections with other users. It has revolutionized the way we function and communicate with each other. Geography is no longer a restriction to the information we can gain or the friends we can make. With the Internet, the world is truly anyone's oyster.

But the Internet can only be beneficial if you really know how to use it and how to take advantage of all it has to offer. Sure, you can perform a quick Google search here and there, but did you know that you can also use the Internet to be a patient and nurse advocate? Nursing doesn't just take place at the bedside. You can make an impact on the lives of patients by using the Internet to its full potential. This may mean using search engines to find information or creating searchable content for the world to see.

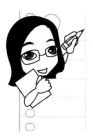

NERDY NOTE

Think outside the box. Don't think about using the Internet only for a singular purpose. Get creative. Sure, you can get information online, but you can also create it for others to access. You have so much nursing knowledge that you could share with the world.

Now, none of this would be possible without search engines and email. One of the greatest Internet-related services and products for users is Google. You know that Google is a big deal when it's routinely being used as a verb and everyone understands the meaning.

In this chapter, I discuss the Internet and Google, plus some additional search engines and how to execute a proper web search. I also dive into some of the services that Google offers that can streamline your life and make you way cooler. Finally, I talk about how to back up your documents and photos online.

SEARCH ENGINE SHOWDOWN

Authority on the Internet is determined by search engines. These web services rank and catalog the content available on the Internet to determine whether it's worthy of being seen. When you type in a search phrase, search engines filter through millions and millions of pages to determine which websites you see. They have the power to show you one page above all others and get your undivided attention. This makes them pretty powerful.

It is important to use a search engine that you can trust. It's an added bonus if the same company that brings you excellent search results also makes other great products. Google, for example, has a multitude of web apps, a browser, and even an operating system (OS). Microsoft, which owns the search engine Bing, is the creator of Windows, Office, and many other products we know and love.

Brand authority means a lot. As consumers, we want to feel comfortable with the products we are using. As nurses, we need to feel confident about the quality of the information we are getting.

You should also know that picking a search engine and service provider is probably going to be a lasting decision, so it's important that you pick the most reliable and easy to use to limit your frustration. It's not so much that you can't use another search engine, but you're likely to get accustomed to certain features and functions. Each search engine operates a little differently, so focusing your efforts on mastering one search engine will help you have a better experience in the long run.

One of the best indications of quality for search engines is consumer adoptions. In other words, the more people who are using it, the better it is. Statowl.com gives percentages of users on the various search engines available. Take a look for yourself to see which search engines others are using:

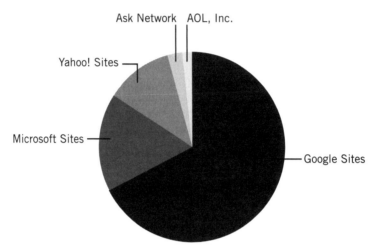

Figure 2.1   Search Engine Rankings in 2013
According to comScore Explicit Core Search Share Report (2013) (figure created by author)

GOOGLE IS GREAT!

As you can see, the majority of people use Google when they are searching the Web. This is important because so many of us rely on information we get online.

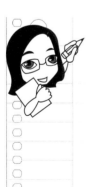

NERDY NOTE

As nurses, we are trusted with protected health information every day. Patients come to us when they are at their most vulnerable, and they trust us to do the right thing. We are given a great amount of trust when they allow us to care for them and have access to their information. This is a great power, and with it comes great responsibility. A web service or search engine should work the same way. It should use the information we give it to improve our experience and then de-identify it when it is shared. This is similar to how nurses must act to ensure that we comply with HIPAA regulations and protect the privacy of our patients.

The Internet would not be what it is today without Google. While this company may have started as a simple search engine, its developers later branched out to provide apps, a web browser, imaging tools, a mobile phone platform, and loads of other tools that can improve your online experience. Google does an excellent job of integrating its many web tools (such as Calendar, Gmail, Tasks, and Drive) into one uniform and fluid experience. The company is also raising the bar for Internet content by increasing the demands for what it considers high-quality to help ensure that only the best content is returned in its search results.

Google integrates many experiences online and allows you to have a much more mobile technological existence.

NERDY NOTE

There is nothing worse than searching for information and being directed to a super spammy website whose primary goal is for you to click on an advertisement. This does nothing to improve the Internet and in general is a huge pain. Google gets this, because it wants to ensure that you get quality search results. Google does not allow spammy websites to appear high in its search rankings, making the Internet a better place overall.

My years of experience with blogging have given me a great deal of insight into how Google operates. If a website attempts to use methods to improve its search standings that are frowned upon by Google, it is quickly yanked from results pages. Keeping up with Google's algorithm (the code that is used to rank websites) is a huge job. The key is that quality always wins, and ultimately the cream rises to the top.

Google is my Best Friend Forever (totally my BFF), and I wouldn't be the nerd I am today without it.

Getting a firm grasp on all the tools that Google offers can really help improve your experience with technology. In this chapter, I focus on its search engine, Chrome, Gmail, Calendar, Drive, Docs, and Maps. These are just a few of the tools that Google offers. Almost all of them play well together and can help automate and simplify your online experiences.

IS YAHOO! FOR YOU?

Yahoo! was once the champion of the Internet and still offers many useful tools. You may be using a Yahoo! product without even realizing it.

Some of the web products and tools that Yahoo! owns include:

+ Flickr

+ Yahoo! Answers

+ Yahoo! Mail

+ Yahoo! Search

Wikipedia (2013) gives a more complete listing of the services and sites owned by Yahoo! I remember when Yahoo! was the primary search engine that was known and trusted. Although many people still use Yahoo! for things like email and Flickr, its search competitors have out-ranked it in user adoption numbers.

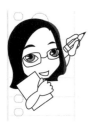

NERDY NOTE

Do you remember those old Yahoo! commercials? I can't shake that pronunciation and singing of the company name at the end of every commercial. Every time I read "Yahoo!" I hear that little singing yodel. Admit it—so do you!

IS BING THE BEST?

Bing is Microsoft's search engine. It is the second-most-used search provider, and many find it easy to use with accurate results. If you're looking for a search engine with a nice visual appeal, then Bing may be right for you.

Something unique about Bing is that Microsoft will actually reward you for using it. Bing Rewards are earned for every search performed on Bing.com. There are also daily rewards that can be earned. Although you won't get rich off the Bing rewards, a few points here and there can really add up. They can be redeemed for a variety of goodies, including gift cards, movie rentals, and more!

If you want to see how Google and Bing compare side by side, you can go to BingItOn. com and in five searches determine which one is right for you.

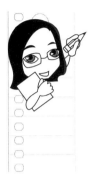

NERDY NOTE

The former professional sweeper (that's someone who enters sweepstakes like a champ) in me really wants to love Bing. Honestly, its search results are pretty good and sometimes even better than Google's. But, my online life revolves around Google services. At this point, I'm pretty much brand loyal to Google, even though in the back of my mind I'm thinking about all the sweet Bing Rewards I could be racking up with every search.

GOOGLE: THE SEARCH ENGINE

When you hear the term "Google," you likely think of the search engine. In fact, the verb "Google" is often used to mean "searching the Web." Google is my go-to search engine because it does an excellent job of ranking websites based upon the quality of their content. The Google algorithm is constantly changing to make sure that it brings back the best results possible. Many webmasters try anything they can to appear in the top rankings of Google. Front-page results can mean big money to many online businesses, so those top spots for many keywords are coveted.

Although you may be finding valuable information on Google, you may not be getting the best results possible. You can get better results out of Google by using Boolean search phrases. Although you may find some results by simply entering a question into Google's search bar, you will get better results if you specify what you are looking for, such as a document type, image, or movie. You can also restrict words or phrases or limit your search to only one website.

You can also use Google to calculate math problems, do conversions, and define words. In fact, many use Google routinely just for spell check, although admittedly this can get you into trouble, because people do spell things incorrectly on the Internet. If you stick with using the definitions, however, you should be safe.

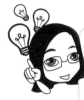

TECH TIP

Bollean search phrases are a very basic sort of search engine logic. It relies on the following symbols to get better search results:

" "	shows exact words or phrases; you can use this multiple times in the same search query
~	shows related words
-	excludes this word from the search
..	shows results within a time range (ex 2008..2012)
site: example.com	only searches pages of the site
filetype: pdf	shows only pdfs in search results

One of the coolest things about Google is that it will automatically suggest search phrases for you. At first this can be a little weird, but it certainly speeds things up. I often scratch my head at how Google seems to know exactly what I'm looking for before I've even looked for it.

GOOGLE CHROME

Google Chrome is an incredibly responsive and useful web browser. It's much faster than Internet Explorer and gives you the ability to download many free add-ons that are called extensions. These extensions can be used to enhance your web experience and can include any number of functions, ranging from fluid Gmail integration to screen capture tools. It is quickly becoming the most popular web browser available.

Speed and reliability are some of the biggest draws of Chrome. It can easily digest complicated code and web designs and spit them back out at you in a seamless and swift manner. Because many websites are actually complex applications, it is important that your go-to web browser be able to handle them without any difficulty. Chrome can load multiple pages and apps at once without a noticeable dip in performance.

As a nurse, you need a fast and efficient web browser that will remember your settings wherever you go. When you create a Google account and sign into Google Chrome, all of your favorite extensions and browsing history are saved in the cloud. If you are researching a topic for a nursing paper or for a presentation at work, then you'll want to be able to access this information any time you have access to a computer and a few moments to work on your research.

If you also take into consideration that Google Docs will take care of your word-processing needs, there is really no reason to use any other web browser.

TECH TIP

"The cloud" is a generic term that relates where documents are stored online. There are many different methods and services that provide this service. You may be familiar with Microsoft SkyDrive, Dropbox, Box, Google Drive, or SugarSync. Basically, these sites allow you to access your files (pictures, music, documents, and more) on any computer with an Internet connection. Some of them even offer smartphone apps!

As part of a clinical assignment in my BSN studies, I used Google Chrome in conjunction with Google Docs when I was doing research about insulin injections requiring two nurses to sign off. I created a folder of favorite websites specific to my research and compiled the information into a document in Google Docs. I also created a shortcut to my document on my toolbar so it was quickly accessible to me when I wanted to work on it. This allowed me to more quickly finish the paper and present the information to the director of nursing at the hospital so that she could present it for consideration to nursing administration.

Chrome is very easy to switch to or start with. If you are already using Internet Explorer or Firefox as your default browser, you can quickly and easily import your existing bookmarks. Chrome also has a very intuitive start page that memorizes the pages you frequent so that they are easily at your fingertips.

NERDY NOTE

I actually use more than one web browser—primarily Chrome, but also Firefox and Internet Explorer if an occasion calls for it.

I have multiple Gmail accounts and get annoyed with having to sign in and out on a single browser, so each browser has a different email address associated with it. Also, some websites are specifically designed to run on Internet Explorer, so I switch over to that when the need arises.

I prefer Chrome because the settings stay with me. Whenever I get a new computer or use a mobile device, I know that once I sign into Google Chrome, the experience will match. All my favorites, extensions, and passwords are securely stored, and it makes owning multiple devices much less cumbersome.

Your Chrome experience is linked to your Google account. This means that any favorites, settings, extensions, and history are saved at the browser level. This really helps ensure that your Internet experience is the same regardless of the device you are using to access the Web.

One of my favorite features of Chrome is its web extensions, browser add-ons that enhance and customize your web-surfing experience. I have downloaded extensions that allow me to take quick notes, save all my passwords, shorten URLs, and share posts on social media sites. There are extensions that instantly let you email a web page or add an appointment to your calendar on your browser bar without navigating to a specific web page or opening another browser window. I also have some ultra-nerdy webmaster extensions that help with blogging. Whatever you like to do online, there is probably an extension to make the experience better.

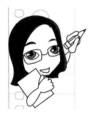

NERDY NOTE
Chrome is available for Mac or PC. It is also available in mobile format for Android and iOS.

Chrome can also be used as a stand-alone OS. It's beefed up a bit and can give you some additional functionality offline and a few other features here and there, but it runs in pretty much the same manner. It incorporates a media player and file browser and is great for people who spend the majority of their time at a computer online. A new Chromebook laptop also comes with 100GB of free storage for 2 years and a small amount of free wireless data. This probably won't be enough for all your Internet needs, so you will need to have some other form of Internet access at home. However, this free mobile wireless data is a great setup for checking email on the go!

If you want to get a notebook computer to help you surf the Web and do little in the way of running traditional Windows-based programs, then a Chromebook might be worth a look. There are some tradeoffs, but a $250 price tag, eight hours of battery life, and Google's support definitely give the Chromebook a little boost in the appeal department. After learning about many of the web apps that Google offers for free, you will understand why it can be easy to switch to the Google Chrome OS.

If you work the nightshift and have hours of downtime, a Chromebook could help you pass that time. You could read up on nursing articles, news, or other interesting topics. They are small and lightweight and have hours of battery life.

CODE CAUTION

Be sure you know your employer's policy on using personal digital devices at work. Many allow them, but some do not. Let your charge nurse know that you are available for help at any time, and don't you dare put your personal device before the wants or needs of your patients.

You should also avoid using social media while on the clock. That sort of activity can be called up later and held against you by your employer and potentially even during legal proceedings.

GMAIL

If I had to pick my most frequented website, application, tool, source of addiction, and personal and business tool, it would have to be Gmail. Although you may have a Hotmail, Yahoo!, or other Internet-provided email account, you have not really experienced how email is supposed to work until you've used Gmail. If you've ever found yourself frustrated or annoyed with email, it's probably because you're not using Gmail.

Email should not be a challenge. It should not take hours to wade through your inbox just to find the messages that are important and relevant to you. Your mail should be automatically sorted based upon filters and labels you've defined or that your mailbox has automatically defined for you. Gmail takes the headache out of email and does it with style.

What's even better about Gmail is that you can use it to check the email of all your accounts at once and from any computer or mobile device. If you go into the settings of Gmail, you can add POP3 email accounts (such as a comcast.net or att.net account), and Gmail will automatically check those mail accounts for you and forward their messages to your Gmail box. This setup does require a little bit of know-how, but once you set it up, it continues to work automatically and can make your life a lot easier. No longer will you be a slave to three or four different websites and applications to check your email; you can check them all in one place and from any device that can access the Internet, including your smartphone.

CODE CAUTION

What is POP3 email? According to Post Office Protocol 3 (POP3; 2007), POP3 is an email protocol in which mail is delivered to your mailbox without retaining a copy on the server. As soon as you download your copy of a message, it is deleted from the mail server. This mimics the way in which the post office operates; when the mail carrier gives you the mail, it's pretty much out of his or her hands.

If you have set your Gmail account access up appropriately, when you reply to emails using the POP3 feature, the recipient sees that the email came from the POP3 email and not your Gmail account. This is useful because it is less confusing for your recipients and ensures that they only know the email address you want them to know.

These instructions explain how to use Gmail for all your email accounts:

1. Create a Gmail account by going to http://gmail.com and clicking the "Create an Account" button on the upper right side of the page.

2. After you have created an account, click on the icon that looks like a gear or cog wheel on the upper right side. Once you click on it, a drop-down menu appears; click on "settings."

3. There is a series of page headings at the top. The fourth one over is "Accounts." Click on it.

4. You now have two areas you need to address: "Send mail as:" and "Check for mail from other accounts (using POP3):".

5. Click on the link beside "Send mail as:" that is labeled "Add another email address you own." Follow the prompts to provide all relevant information.

6. Click on the link beside "Check for mail from other accounts (using POP3):" that is labeled "Add a POP3 mail account you own." As with step 5, follow the prompts.

7. Complete any verification processes that Google asks. Usually for sending email, Google wants to send a verification code via text message. This is just to prevent spammers.

8. Repeat this process for as many email addresses as you have.

9. It's as simple as that! Now you've got all your email accounts in one place and can send and reply to any messages without having to jump around to multiple apps and web locations.

TECH TIP

When you add an email account to Gmail, it is going to ask for your password. Google is safe and secure, so you can feel confident about providing your password. Remember, this is your email account, so only you can access the information stored within it.

Another awesome thing about Gmail is that it works great with a smartphone. Whether you choose an iPhone or an Android device, Gmail and your account settings will integrate with it, including your contacts, your calendar appointments, and your settings. You can also choose to integrate your notes from your phone into Google as well. It uses IMAP technology, which means that anything you delete, edit, send, or reply to on your phone will be the same when you check it on a web browser. This makes staying current with your email on the go easy, because you don't have to worry about checking and deleting the same mail twice.

You may be able to access your work email from home. Check your employer's policy to find out whether this is possible or allowed. You may need to sign a form to have this ability. You will also need to know which mail server your employer uses.

On an Android device or iPhone, the setup is fairly simple. You will need to go to settings and mail/exchange accounts. After that, you will need to add an account. Fill in your user name, password, and the mail server information that you got from your manager or the IT department.

If you run into a snag getting this set up, my best advice for you is to Google it! I've already mentioned how much information is available on Google, and I promise you that more than a few tutorials are devoted to setting up mail on smartphones.

If you're concerned about viruses and spam, then Gmail's got you covered with its excellent spam-detection technology. It also automatically screens your messages for viruses and other malware and will indicate whether it thinks it's safe to open an email or follow the links within it.

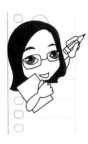

NERDY NOTE

Integrating your phone's notes and contacts into Google is an excellent way to make sure they are backed up.

When you set up your mail account on your phone, you will have the option to integrate your notes and calendar. Make sure you select it.

Gmail also automatically saves the addresses of people you email frequently in your contact list. You can use an extension like Rapportive to show additional details about the contacts in the sidebar of the page, such as their social media accounts and latest tweets. This is a great way to easily see where you can find out more about someone you have been emailing.

Setting up Rapportive or any other Chrome extension is supereasy. Just Google "Rapportive extension," and the first link should be to the Google Chrome extension. Click on "add to Chrome." Follow any prompts and authorize any apps it asks for. It's not going to spam anyone or anything.

TECH TIP

The Rapportive extension is also available in Firefox and Safari.

You should know, however, that Gmail and other Google apps are designed to work best in Google Chrome. You wouldn't want to put low-fat cream cheese in a cheesecake, would you? It would probably get the job done and taste OK, but you'd completely ruin the integrity of a good cheesecake!

GOOGLE CALENDAR

The Google Calendar web app is easy to use and integrates seamlessly with Gmail. Like Gmail, it can easily integrate into your smartphone. This makes keeping track of your day-to-day activities, work schedule, and important events a breeze. It also makes it easy to update your calendar on the go.

A really cool feature of Google Calendar is its ability to send appointment requests and event invitations, especially for group activities. If you are on a nursing or hospital committee at work that will be meeting several times, it is great to plot out all the appointments on a

Google Calendar that can be shared and updated by other team members. The same concept applies if you are in school doing a group project; sharing an entire calendar can really help your team stay on track with important deadlines.

Scheduling on Google Calendar is simple to do in a computer-based browser or on a smartphone. You need to have a Google account with Gmail already set up and then browse on over to google.com/calendar and click "create." Fill out the details for your appointment; you can even choose to share this appointment with others.

In addition, Google Calendar is a great way to keep track of your busy family's activities. You can share appointments with your family to make sure everyone is aware of the schedule. You can even create separate calendars to track different things. Here are some types of calendars you might create.

One neat thing that I recently helped a colleague of mine set up was an appointment calendar for his aging parents' medical appointments and medication reminders. They created a Gmail account for him and set it up on their phone and his. They were able to add appointments to the calendar on his phone through their own smartphone simply by making sure they selected his calendar when making the appointments. His calendar was automatically updated without his having to do a thing.

Google Calendar is also great for:

> ✛ **Bills.** You can plot the dates that your bills are due and approximate amounts owed. It's also a good idea to put your paycheck schedule on there so that you can keep your finances in line.

> ✛ **Family activities.** If your children or grandchildren are active in sports, music, or any other extracurricular activity, tracking their appointments is vital. You wouldn't want to miss a big swim team meet or choir performance.

> ✛ **Work schedules.** If your schedule changes or you have specific appointments to keep for work, you might want to separate this calendar from general use.

> ✛ **Personal.** This calendar is great to keep track of personal appointments, events you want to remember, and maybe even date nights.

> ✛ **Nursing continuing education (CE).** If your state requires CE hours, you will want to make sure that you keep up when you have to take the courses. This is a great way to keep track of when you have education sessions scheduled as well as making notes for yourself on what you've already done.

> ✛ **Nursing license.** Having a calendar with important nursing dates can remind you when you need to renew your license or different certifications you hold.

Google is the king of Internet searches, and it's no different when it comes to your calendar. You can easily search your scheduled and past appointments for specific words. You can also use this feature on public calendars.

When you create a calendar, you have the option to make it public or private. If you have initially created a private calendar and later want to make it public, you can do so in the calendar settings. Here's how:

1. After you have gone to the Google Calendar page, you should see a list of all the calendars you've created.

2. Click on the arrow beside the name and then choose "calendar settings."

3. Scroll down until you see a link titled "Change sharing settings" under Calendar Address. Click on it.

4. You then have the option of making the calendar public and/or sharing it with specific email addresses.

If your nursing career requires you to travel, Google Calendar can make your life a little easier. You can integrate Google Maps directly into your calendar to help you better plan your trip and get directions to your appointments. This application is also helpful if you are planning an event, because you can use Google Calendar to send out invitations. What better way to make sure your guests know how to find you?

GOOGLE DRIVE

Google Drive is Google's answer to cloud computing. It is an online file storage tool that can synchronize documents and files on your computer. It's also integrated with Google Docs, which is a group of productivity tools, including word processing, spreadsheets, presentations, forms, and drawings. Like most of Google's services, Google Drive is provided for free along with Google Docs. You can choose to upgrade your storage limits for a nominal annual fee.

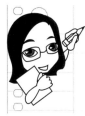

NERDY NOTE

What is the cloud? It basically is a way to store your documents remotely to reduce the threat of loss on your personal system and to allow you to access them from other computers or mobile devices.

Synchronizing your computer to the cloud has several benefits. First and foremost, it protects your data by backing it up to a remote location. Secondly, it allows you access to your files while you are on the go. Third, it's automated, which takes most of the potential user error out of the process. Finally, most experts agree that storing data in the cloud is more secure than storing it on an unprotected hard drive.

Depending on your role in a hospital, you may or may not have access to email and the hospital file network. Many organizations are leery of putting patient information in the cloud due to HIPAA concerns, and you should be as well.

If you have created a custom template for taking reports at shift change, then the cloud would be an excellent way to store it. This way you could make sure you have access to it at any time and at any location, thus eliminating the need to store the file directly on your employer's computer or network.

GOOGLE DOCS

For many people, Google Docs is quickly becoming their go-to resource for creating documents. Many find that they don't even need to fork over hundreds of dollars for Microsoft Office anymore, because Google Docs meets their needs. Although Microsoft Office definitely has its strong points, for most average users, Google Docs more than meets their needs for the fantastic price of free! Yep, that's right—FREE!

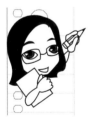

NERDY NOTE
Google Chrome is the recommended browser for using Google Docs. It runs much more smoothly, and the applications are designed to run on that browser.

Five types of files can be created using Google Docs. Each of these is similar to software that many of us routinely pay for. It's also worth noting that Google Docs works anywhere with a web connection, so you don't have to be concerned about making sure you have your computer with you or that the machine you're using has the software installed. You just hop on the Internet and bounce on over to http://drive.google.com. Sign in to your Google account and get to writing, calculating, or whatever strikes your fancy.

Most health care organizations will probably stay away from Google Docs for reports and data that contain protected health information (PHI). However, if you deal with vendors or other outside organizations, then Google Docs is a good way to share information that does not contain PHI.

Table 2.1   Equivalent programs between Google Docs and Microsoft Office

GOOGLE DOCS	Document	Spreadsheet	Presentation	Form	Drawing
MICROSOFT OFFICE	Word	Excel	PowerPoint	N/A	Paint

If you're working on a project with multiple nurses at a hospital for a committee or project, then you might want to suggest using Google Docs as a collaborative tool. It's a great way for multiple people to update the same document and get notifications when changes are made.

After you have created the document you wish to share, it's easy to get others in on the action. With the document open in your browser, you can click on "share" on the upper right side. You can then add people to collaborate on or view the document by email address, and you can adjust their individual document privileges in the same screen.

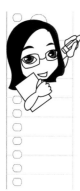

NERDY NOTE

If you don't want to pay the money for Microsoft Office but still want a piece of traditional software to create office documents, you might want to consider free software called OpenOffice.

OpenOffice is an office suite that includes free versions of programs similar to Microsoft Word, Excel, and PowerPoint. You can download OpenOffice at www.openoffice.org/download/. It offers a different user experience that lacks some of Microsoft's bells and whistles, but most people find that it gets the job done.

GOOGLE DOCUMENT

Google Document functions like Microsoft Word. This is useful for creating documents primary composed of text that doesn't require any calculations. The developers give you a very robust group of tools that should be familiar to you if you use other Google web apps. When using Google Document, you will notice that there is far less clutter on the screen than in Microsoft Word. You have fewer options on your menu than you might have in Microsoft Word, but most people find that they have all they need. You also have the ability to embed images and drawings in your documents to spruce up their visual appeal. Overall, Google Document is an excellent word-processing tool that could easily replace a desktop word-processing program.

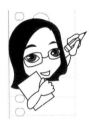

NERDY NOTE

Google Docs really does a lot of the work for you. For instance, it automatically saves your document every 3 to 4 minutes.

Ways nurses can use Google Docs include:

+ Collaborating on a nursing committee

+ Sharing documents with vendors or organizations outside their employers

+ Creating web-based presentations that only need a browser to load

+ Saving report templates to access them anywhere

TECH TIP

Use F11 on your keyboard to switch your web browser to full screen. This will hide the menus and address bars at the top of your screen and give you a lot of document real estate to work with.

GOOGLE SPREADSHEET

Google Spreadsheet is a steadfast competitor to Microsoft Excel. Its formatting features are fairly similar to those in Google Document, with the addition of spreadsheet-specific icons and menus. This is an excellent tool to use for budgets, numbered lists, or anything that requires any sort of calculation. Google Spreadsheet can handle pretty much everything that most Excel users might need.

Google Spreadsheet can be useful for tracking personal financial details and data that require calculation. It can also be helpful if you need to share information outside your organization.

If you are responsible for compiling information that contains PHI, then a personal Google Docs account is not a good choice. You should default to Microsoft Excel and use internal devices that store the information on your hospital's secure network.

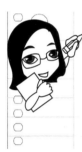

NERDY NOTE

Google Spreadsheet automatically saves every time you change a cell. If you're like me and often multitask/get multidistracted, then this is huge help. No longer do I have to be bothered with hitting the save button and wasting valuable seconds and exerted energy. In fact, Google Docs doesn't even include a save icon. Admittedly, that blew my mind a little, but you'll get used to it after a while.

GOOGLE PRESENTATION

Google Presentation is a very basic slideshow creation web app. If you are a fan of Power-Point and are familiar with some of its higher-end functions, you might be a bit disappointed, because at this point, Google Presentation is limited. One of the most noticeable absences is charts and graphs. For many people, using PowerPoint to create presentations, charts, and graphs is a necessity, so this barebones approach is unfortunate. However, if you just want to create a basic presentation in an easy-to-use system, then Google Presentation will meet your needs.

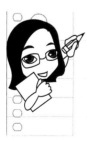

NERDY NOTE

Google does a great job of keeping the look of its apps clean and consistent.

The location for editing a document, an email, or a spreadsheet is uniform. If you learn to use the functions in one Google app or service, you should have no trouble finding and using them in another.

GOOGLE FORM

Google Form doesn't really have a Microsoft counterpart. It is a great tool to use for collecting information and storing it in a centralized location. You can create a "form" and give the link to individuals to complete. The form creates a series of data fields that, when completed, appear in a spreadsheet. If you are taking a poll, collecting orders, or making a mailing list, Google Form is a great tool.

If you're looking for a way to compile data for research, then Google Form has you covered. It's an excellent tool for clinical research or collecting other data, automatically incorporating it into an organized spreadsheet.

One of the nicest features is that the look and feel of Google Form are customizable, so you can really make it your own. This is helpful when you want to create a survey that is professional and elicits answers from a respondent.

Google Form can be embedded within an existing website. On a nursing blog, you can use Google Form to survey readers regarding a particular topic. This is useful if you are researching how many nurses have experienced bullying in the workplace, for example, or what nurses think is the proper patient-to-nurse ratio.

After you create a Google Form, you receive an embed code. If you are editing a page in HMTL, just insert this embed code in the location where you want the form to appear. If you don't know how to edit HTML, you can provide the code to your webmaster for inclusion on the site.

GOOGLE DRAWING

Google Drawing is an excellent Microsoft Paint replacement. You can insert images, add text, draw freehand, add shapes, fill colors, and so on. The drawings you create can be saved as a JPG, PNG, SVG, or PDF and posted on the Web or inserted into a Google Document or Presentation. It's simple but useful if you want to create an image and don't need any super-complex tools.

If you are organizing a clinical study, you can use Google Drawing to prepare graphics or signage you might need. If you are counting on nurses to keep track of certain pieces of documentation, a visually stimulating reminder is helpful when posted in various places around the nurses station.

TECH TIP

Google Drawing works great with a touch-screen computer.

Because it is a drawing application, you can use freeform drawing to customize your image. Your finger interacts with a screen in the same way that scrolling or clicking a mouse does. It's also just a lot more fun than using a traditional mouse.

Google Docs and Drive are a revolution in cloud computing. When I was in nursing school, I would have loved a word processor that saved all my papers in the cloud so that I could work on them when I had a few hours free between classes. This is just one of the many forms of technology that are making life easier every day.

As I mentioned earlier, Google Drive and Docs are free and include 5GB of free storage. Most people find this is more than enough to save all their documents. If you are going to be using Google's photo service, Picasa, then it is worth noting that this file storage amount does not change. Photos are usually very large files and consequently are space hogs. If you plan on storing all your photos on Google Drive or Picasa, then you may want to consider paying for additional storage.

Picasa is a photo-editing and storage tool. You can enhance your images and also share them with friends or family. You can also use a service like Picasa to catalog images you are using for research or as part of a presentation.

TECH TIP

If you want to back up your photos online, you should probably invest in additional storage.

Many people choose to back up images on external hard drives, thumb drives, CDs, or DVDs. I personally do not recommend these options, because the files can become corrupted or the storage system can become unusable. If this occurs, then your images are lost forever.

Backing up in the cloud ensures that your files are stored in multiple locations and are much more secure.

GOOGLE MAPS

Google Maps is a web app that allows you to use maps in many different ways. You can find directions and print them directly from a computer. A mobile app gives you directions right on your smartphone. Another cool feature of Google Maps is Streetview. You can actually type in an address and see a photographic image of the area as if you were standing on the street. Many of these are 360-degree views, allowing you to virtually explore an area. When you are planning a home hospice visit, Google Maps is a great tool to let you know exactly where you are going and what to look for.

TECH TIP

To get the best results with any of Google's web apps, it is recommended that you use Google Chrome. As I mentioned before, Google designs its apps and products to work best in the Chrome browser. If you want to ensure a fluid experience, Google Chrome is the way to go.

ARE YOU GOOD TO GO ON GOOGLE?

By now you should have a little more background on search engines and be able to execute an accurate Google search. You should be able to integrate other email accounts into your Gmail account. You should feel more comfortable using Google apps and have a greater appreciation for how you can use them. You also know how to install a Chrome extension and how to create public or private Google calendars.

Whew! We accomplished a lot in this chapter. Are you ready for more?

REFERENCES

Flosi, S. (2013, 12 April). comScore releases March 2013 U.S. search engine rankings. comScore. Retrieved from http://www.comscore.com/Insights/Press_Releases/2013/4/comScore_Releases_March_2013_U.S._Search_Engine_Rankings

List of Yahoo!-owned sites and services. (2013, 16 May). In Wikipedia. Retrieved from http://en.wikipedia.org/wiki/List_of_Yahoo!-owned_sites_and_services

Rouse, M. (2007, March). POP3 (Post Office Protocol 3). SearchExchange. Retrieved from http://searchexchange.techtarget.com/definition/POP3

3

SOCIAL MEDIA: THE EASY, FAST, AND FUN WAY TO COMMUNICATE

The Internet has revolutionized the way we communicate with each other and whom we define as friends. We are swiftly becoming a global community and have opportunities to network with almost anyone in the world. Geographic location has become largely insignificant, and entire social communities exist solely online.

Although using social media is a fun and efficient way to connect with friends and family, social networking is also great for your career. If you are passionate about nursing, then increasing your nursing knowledge while communicating with other nurses online will be both pleasurable and potentially even financially beneficial.

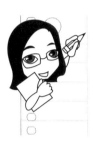

NERDY NOTE
Did you ever think about the fact that social media removes limitations and costs from worldwide communication?

I have friends in Minnesota whom I see and hear from more often than the friends who live just a few blocks down the street.

Before we go much further, we should probably define social media:

> Social media is a collective term referring to interactions among groups of people online where information and types of media are created and shared.

These online groups are often referred to as communities and can be based on any number of ideas, principles, or common interests, whether personal or professional. You can use social media to get a good laugh or to spread a message about how hospital administrators can improve their treatment of bedside nurses. The choice is yours and truly limited only by what you can imagine.

Social media gives you the power to change the world, if you choose to do so. You can spread a positive message and bring attention to issues that might otherwise go unnoticed. You no longer need to rely on traditional mass media outlets when you're trying to make the world pay attention to a topic. Your message can go viral based on its merit alone.

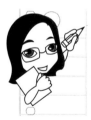

NERDY NOTE
Do you have an idea to share? Are passionate about a particular topic? Social media is a great way to connect with others who share the same interests and goals!

With great power comes great responsibility. When you use social media, you should be aware of what you are saying and to whom you are saying it. Anything written on the Internet might as well be written in stone. Anything you say or do can be traced back to you and remain attached to your name forever. Think twice or perhaps even three times before making comments on a topic, whether they are positive or negative.

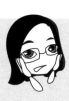

CODE CAUTION

This online permanence includes photos!

The media have shown many examples of nurses and nursing students taking inappropriate photographs and then sharing them online. Something as simple as a picture taken at the nurse's station can be inappropriate if it contains PHI. Cameras can catch those tiny details, and when the images are expanded, they are often legible. This is a HIPAA violation and can incur a huge fine!

There are also examples of x-rays and other patient images that have been circulated online. It is completely inappropriate to share this sort of information under any circumstances.

Remember how your mother always told you that if you couldn't say anything nice, then you shouldn't say anything at all? These rules apply in social media. If you want to provide criticism, that is one thing, but being habitually negative is not recommended. No one wants to be friends with a bully, online or off.

Although it's unfortunate, bullying exists in the nursing profession. Social media has the potential to make matters worse. If a colleague is bullying you at work, on Facebook, or via any other platform, you need to let your manager know. Whether you are on the clock or off, this sort of behavior isn't acceptable and should not be tolerated.

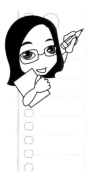

NERDY NOTE

Use social media for good instead of evil.

I've read many nursing blogs whose authors include a great deal of profanity and talk negatively about their patients and other nurses. This approach does nothing to elevate them or the nursing profession. It could also come back to haunt them if their colleagues or patients were to find identifiable information within these postings.

Some of the most familiar and commonly used social networking sites are Facebook, Twitter, Google+, and LinkedIn. These large social networking websites are actually sophisticated applications that provide many ways for users to connect and share ideas, experiences, images, and links. Each site has its own strengths and weaknesses, and many individuals feel strongly about using one over another.

NERDY NOTE

This Nerdy Nurse prefers Twitter.

Although I use many social media platforms, Twitter has struck me as the best. It's easy to craft a short message, and the brevity of 140 characters ensures that you have to be succinct in what you say. I find that I meet more people with common interests on Twitter because Twitter is where you go to meet people you want to be friends with, whereas Facebook is where you go to add people to your friend list whom you may not like but feel obligated to add. Chances are that if you haven't added people you know on Facebook, they might think that you do not like them. This just adds to the level of drama that can be associated with Facebook.

Twitter creates far less drama, because even though you may know people you follow, you probably don't know most of them, so none of your friends or family should seriously be offended if you don't follow them or reply to each of their tweets. As you likely already know, on Facebook, there's a chance that they might. Been there, done that, got the proverbial T-shirt.

Twitter is also where you go to talk to the world. Facebook is more personal and intimate (if you have your privacy settings configured correctly). Twitter is meant to facilitate an open conversation where people who aren't friends with you can still easily interact with you. It really helps open up conversations.

Most people have a favorite social networking site, but they all serve unique purposes. For example, Facebook is great for connecting with family and friends. Twitter is ideal for connecting with celebrities and brands and sharing random thoughts and articles. Google+ allows you to connect with groups that share a common interest. LinkedIn is best-suited for connecting with professionals who share your career passions. Although many of these functions overlap onto other social networking sites, many people believe that to get a more fully rounded social media experience, it is best to use several social networking sites for different purposes.

In this chapter, I discuss various forms of social media and how you can use them to further your nursing career and the nursing profession. I provide a little insight regarding why you should be involved with social media and go over the differences among a blog, a forum, and a social network. And if you have a Facebook account but aren't sure why or are considering deleting it altogether, then this chapter is going to take you for a ride.

After reading this chapter, you should have a better understanding of:

✦ Facebook

✦ Twitter

✦ Google+

✦ LinkedIn

✦ Forums

✦ Blogs

WHY NURSES NEED TO BE INVOLVED IN SOCIAL MEDIA

If you can gain one thing from being involved with social media as a nurse, it's community. Over the years, the one constant in social media is that everyone is trying to make a connection with someone. No one wants to feel alone in the world.

There are many moments in our nursing careers that leave us feeling very isolated. As a new nurse, you may often be far away from your nursing school friends while trying to figure out how to be a successful nurse and how to navigate the politics of health care. Wouldn't it be nice to know there was a place you could go where someone else has already gone through the experiences you are facing? Wouldn't it be nice to know that you are not alone in your struggle to make these adjustments?

You can talk with your friends and family about the issues you face at work, but unless they've been in the same situations, they just really won't completely understand. And as helpful as it is to talk about your experiences and how they make you feel, what you'd really like to know is how to handle these unique nursing situations and what others have done in the same scenarios. Fear not—social media has the answers.

When I first started blogging about nursing, I wrote about my experiences with lateral violence. I wrote about the pain I experienced and the difficulties I was facing because my colleagues were treating me as less than. I researched bullying in nursing and wrote articles about how the ongoing issue affected patient care and techniques to combat it. What I found through this process is that I was far from alone in my struggles with lateral violence. And even though I wouldn't have wished my experience on anyone else in the world, some small part of me was thankful to know that I wasn't alone.

Bullying elevated the stress of nursing to a monumental level. It got to the point where I was so alienated at work that I had no one to talk to, turn to, or ask for help with patient needs. They say you can't nurse on an island, but for more than a year of my nursing career, that's what it felt like I was doing.

I was alone, stressed, tired, and feeling so confused. I was unsure about my career choice and even more unsure about remaining in health care and nursing in general. Was this what nursing was going to be like? Were there more people out there like this? Was this behavior going to follow me everywhere I went?

When it became too much for me, I turned to social media. I started talking to others about the topic. I started researching other examples and found that I wasn't alone. I started writing, sharing, and connecting with other nurses who had similar experiences. This gave me the confidence and strength I needed to carry on and keep on nursing.

We all need to have connections with others who share similar experiences to us. Sometimes we cannot find those people in "real life." Thankfully, we now have alternative means to locate individuals with similar interests and experiences to our own. Social media can connect us to others with similar goals and passions.

As nurses, we need to take a proactive approach to shaping the future of our profession. By using social media, we can get large groups of nurses to weigh in on pressing issues. We can create meaningful conversations that can promote positive change in the nursing profession. But we need more nurses involved to do this. We need you to get online and become a part of the social media nursing community so that you can help shape the future of our profession.

CONNECTING WITH THE NURSING COMMUNITY ONLINE

There are many communities and ways to connect with other nurses online. LinkedIn offers groups. Twitter includes lists and Twitter chats. Google+ has communities. Facebook provides pages and groups. These various groups may be generalized and include all types of nursing or may be grouped into specialties. You can also visit websites called forums, which are social networks completely devoted to a common theme or interest. Another option is to visit nurse-operated blogs where you can read and comment on web content created by other nurses. Regardless of the nurse running the blog, one thing that seems to be fairly consistent with nurses no matter where we live or what we specialize in is that we get other nurses.

Within 5 minutes, you could probably think of at least 10 issues that are present in the nursing world. Nursing shortages, nurse-to-patient ratios, lateral violence, level of pay, inability to take breaks, nursing's image in the media, and fear of being a good patient advocate are just a few of the issues that come to mind. It's important to not silently sit by and allow ourselves to be victims of these issues. It's up to us to change the culture and correct the issues, but no one nurse can do it alone. By uniting online, we can start discussions about important issues affecting our profession.

FACEBOOK

More than one billion registered users have Facebook accounts. If you're even remotely involved in technology, it's likely that you're on Facebook or have been at some point. Although the pages of Facebook often display more dramas and tragedies than a bad soap opera, you can leverage its power in some really useful ways to grow as a nurse.

Facebook groups, pages, and chats are some tools that the website offers to get conversations started. These can be used in conjunction to reach larger or smaller audiences, depending on the purpose of the conversation. Many popular nursing websites, blogs, and forums also have a Facebook presence.

If you are discussing an intimate issue, then a chat or group message allows only the people invited to see the information. It also ensures that all communication has equal weight. However, if the conversation involves more than just a few people, then a chat can be difficult to manage.

FACEBOOK PAGES

Facebook pages are great ways to connect with nurses. Many nursing websites also have dedicated Facebook pages with thousands of fans. These pages often post new content daily, and you can interact with the page owners and other fans via comments and likes. You can also post your own messages to the page walls, but these may get overlooked, because most fans only permit updates from the page owners to show in their newsfeed. These are still great ways to connect with other nurses, but if you have something to say to a large group and you aren't the page owner, your message may get lost.

FACEBOOK GROUPS

One of the best ways to connect with other nurses is Facebook groups. Groups can allow you to create smaller networks among your existing friends and separate their conversations from the rest of what you see on Facebook. Groups can be open, private, or secret. Depending on the setting you choose, your group may appear in search listings or may only be available to those with an invitation.

Facebook groups are some of the best ways to connect with other nurses. Groups offer many resources that enhance social networking. One great example of this is the "Docs" feature, which allows you to create documents that can be shared and even edited by the group. This is useful for sharing agendas, updates to nursing legislature, or perhaps a listing of Congressional representatives' email addresses and phone numbers.

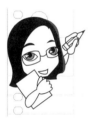

NERDY NOTE

Sometimes the "Docs" feature can be a little confusing. A better alternative is to use Google Docs, which we discussed in the previous chapter.

Many Facebook groups and pages allow you to connect with other nurses and share ideas, get informed about the latest issues, and broaden your nursing horizons. What you get out of Facebook is really up to you. If you're willing to put a little time and effort into it, then it can be a powerful communication tool that connects you with a community of passionate and opinionated nurses.

I've found that smaller Facebook groups can really be beneficial to discuss common interests or to work toward a common goal. I am a part of a Facebook group with other nurse bloggers, and we use this group to share opportunities with others in the group. Opportunities for nurse bloggers vary, but they might include a referral to a business that is looking for content experts, a freelance writing job, or another opportunity to grow their business. Being a part of this community has helped me bounce ideas off other members and get support when I needed it.

FACEBOOK GAMES

But don't let all the networking you can do with other nurses stop you from having a little non-nursing fun as well! You can connect with your family and close and personal friends to share pictures, your thoughts, or your location. You can also like your favorite businesses, brands, celebrities, and websites to get updates on their current happenings and upcoming events.

Facebook also includes many fun and challenging games that can keep you occupied for hours on end. These are a great way to relax and relieve stress. They are also a little more fun than other games, because many let you play with your friends and family. Although some argue that such games are a waste of time, I truly believe that you need moments to unwind now and then, and Facebook games provide an excellent opportunity to do this.

Although I try to stay away from Facebook games, because they can be extremely time consuming, I do enjoy playing Candy Crush, which is a fun little game that integrates with Facebook. You move candies around to align them in patterns and crush them. You also have to achieve certain goals to advance through each level in the game. It may sound a bit silly—and, well, it is—but that doesn't make it any less fun!

Many Facebook games actually make you use your brain, including such word games as Words With Friends and Scramble With Friends. You can feel a little less guilty about playing these games because they are great for your mind. It's also fun to play these because you are competing with your friends to determine who is the best wordsmith.

Many strategy-based games are also fun to play. Whether it's Farmville or The Sims, the games largely operate the same but with varying goals and responsibilities. They are equally silly, but once you get started, it can be difficult to stop playing. They are as addicting as any other habit, and I've even had a few Facebook game interventions in my own life, but that's a story for another day.

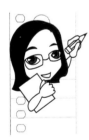

NERDY NOTE

Many Facebook games have a smartphone app counterpart, which allows you to continue your progress in the game while you are on the go.

This is probably not a good idea if you are already addicted to a Facebook game . . . or is it?

TWITTER

Twitter is a social network that is often misunderstood. When I was first introduced to Twitter, I really thought it was pointless. It took a little while for me to get what it was all about and how it was different from—and in many ways better than—other social media sites. Twitter is my personal favorite social media platform, and many of its users feel the same way.

When I first got started with Twitter, it was overwhelming, and I felt like I was talking to no one. That's probably because in the beginning, I was. I had to learn to put an @ in front of a user name if I wanted that person to see it. I also didn't know then that a person has to be following you before you can send him or her a direct (private) message.

I also totally didn't get hashtags, which are a large part of the Twitter community. I didn't understand that a hashtag could be used to categorize a status update as well as to provide the punch line of a joke. But the more I used Twitter, the more I began to understand that you can't just dip your toes in the Twitter water—you have to dive into the Twitter ocean.

TECH TIP

A hashtag is a word or words starting with a # that are grouped together and represent a common theme. Some examples are #Nurses, #HCSM (Health Care Social Media), #FF (Follow Friday), #NursingJobs, and #NursingSchool.

They can signify all sorts of things. For example, the hashtag #HCSM is used when someone wants to show that a topic might be of importance to the Health Care Social Media community. The hashtag #FF is a quick way for tweeters to identify fellow Twitter users whom they think you should follow. This often happens on a Friday, but not always.

The defining characteristic of Twitter is that it limits your "tweets" (Twitter's version of Facebook's "status update") to 140 characters. The brevity of the tweets forces you to be thoughtful about the words you use to convey your message. You can't ramble on endlessly. You have to get to the point.

One of the best ways I can describe the difference between Facebook and Twitter is that Facebook is usually the way to connect with people you actually know but may not always like, while Twitter is how you can connect with people you don't know personally but do like. Twitter is where you can go to expand your social networking horizon and connect with celebrities, brands, and others who share common interests.

Twitter is less complicated than Facebook in many ways. It doesn't have games or groups, but there are ways to categorize the people you follow. You can follow individuals and categorize them by common interests in lists. You can search by user names, keywords, or hashtags. You can even dig in deeper and search for keywords in user bios or in a specific user's tweets.

TWITTER CHATS AND HASHTAGS

Twitter chats are usually hourlong sessions of discussion focusing on predefined topics chosen by moderators. These are often organized by bloggers, businesses, or other social media enthusiasts. These chats are a great way to meet other Twitter users with whom you share a common interest, to find people to follow, and to have others follow you. Any tweet that should be considered part of the chat conversation should include the hashtag specific to the chat. A popular Twitter chat for nurses is #RNchat. The hashtag #HCSM is also very popular and stands for "Health Care Social Media." The hashtag for the Twitter chat is decided beforehand by the TweetChat organizer. If you want to be involved in the chat, make sure you include the hashtag in your comments. It you don't, others won't see your tweets.

Twitter chats are fast-paced and usually have a very interactive audience. Many find it helpful to use a third-party service, such as TweetDeck or TweetChat, to get the most out of a Twitter chat. These services offer some added functionality, such as automatically updating, automatically including the hashtag, and many other useful features. You can also search for the relevant hashtags after the fact to be sure you are following those in the chat whom you found interesting or responding to those whom you thought made relevant or irrelevant points.

The hashtag #FF is probably one of the most popular. You can use this hashtag along with the @username of people you follow whom you think others should also follow. It's a good way to give recognition to people you follow whom you think are interesting, funny, or making a difference online.

TWITTER—MORE THAN JUST A PLAYGROUND OF FUN

Although many feel that Twitter is just an excuse for narcissists to have their mundane ramblings acknowledged (and trust me, there is plenty of that!), Twitter is so much more than that to so many people.

As I mentioned previously, I was bullied earlier in my nursing career and used social media as a coping mechanism. My social media platform of choice was Twitter, and it was instrumental in helping me cope with a difficult work situation. When I felt I had no one else in the world to talk to, I had Twitter. I had a community of nurses and non-nurses alike who sympathized with my situation and were disgusted by what I was going through. I had friends all over the world who talked to me on my lunch break and laughed at my corny jokes. At a time in my life when I was at my lowest, Twitter helped lift me up and make me feel like what I said mattered.

I've also used Twitter to help spread nursing humor and positive nursing initiatives. Twitter is a great way to share news and images with a broad community. If Facebook is the proverbial watercooler, then Twitter is the soapbox. You can reach a lot of people who will share your message with their audiences and reach greater numbers of people very quickly.

You can also be a "man on the street" and give updates on events you witness. People flock to Twitter to share images of events they see and leave commentary. It's a good way to keep others informed and to stay informed yourself.

The potential to move news quickly among a large audience is extremely helpful during natural disasters and other major news events. You can get information about events much quicker on Twitter than many other news mechanisms. In fact, many news organizations check Twitter to get information on events as they are happening. The news organizations then share this information with their own audience. I'm sure you've seen your local news anchors referencing Twitter a time or two. It's pretty amazing to think that you could help others by tweeting, but you can.

NERDY NOTE

If you're a nurse who has ever felt bullied or even just ignored, Twitter can be an outlet like no other. You can discuss your frustrations with current nursing issues that you see every day. You can ask questions and share quotes. You can reference that you are a nurse on social media without a threat, but you always have to be cautious of what you say. Your words are forever tied to you and your profession, and you need to make sure that they present the image that you want. You also have to be conscious of HIPAA guidelines and not disclose any identifying patient information.

My best advice for you is to never talk about anything specific that can be tied back to a particular event, patient encounter, or even your health care organization. Write about nursing issues and participate in the conversations, but don't provide any ammunition that could be used against you.

If you are going to write publicly as a nurse, then make sure that anything you write could be read aloud in front of your boss and a human resources officer. If you can't do this, then you probably shouldn't write it.

LINKEDIN

LinkedIn is the social network for professionals. A LinkedIn account is basically a digital resume, but you can enhance it by increasing your connections. LinkedIn also gives you the ability to receive recommendations and endorsements from those with whom you are connected. These endorsements can give a boost to your profile and improve your image in the eyes of potential employers.

If you are a job seeker, you can use LinkedIn to enhance your search. You can seek out connections of hiring managers. You can ask current or former employers to post recommendations on your profile. Your connections can also add endorsements related to your skill set. You can go to different groups and answer questions to demonstrate your knowledge level. And you can also see who has been looking at your profile, which may give you some insight regarding how visible your profile is.

Connections are the people whom you have invited to be a part of your network or who have asked to join your network. They are basically the LinkedIn version of Facebook "friends." Being on LinkedIn, in the digital age, just makes sure that you are seen. If you are competing for a nursing job against other applicants who may be more technologically savvy than you, then your name and face may not be seen by recruiters and hiring managers as often. Say, for example, that you go to an interview with a nurse manager or other hiring manager, and you want to make sure that you stay on this person's mind. Inviting the interviewer to connect with you on LinkedIn is a great way to keep your name on the tip of his or her tongue and hopefully at the top of the list of potential applicants. LinkedIn recommendations can really help set your profile apart from others. A recommendation indicates that someone thought enough of you and your performance to take the time to write about it. In today's fast-paced world, this is no small feat. Glowing recommendations can help give personal insights into what makes you a valuable employee. If at all possible, you should ask any bosses or colleagues you feel comfortable with to leave a recommendation for you on LinkedIn.

ENDORSEMENTS

Endorsements are a quick and easy way for your connections to weigh in on your skills and expertise. By simply clicking on a skill, they can add their endorsement of your knowledge of this skill to your profile. The more endorsements you have for a skill, the higher it ranks in your profile. It also shows the images of those endorsers next to the skill. Basically, those people are vouching for your skills. An endorsement is much faster and easier to give than a recommendation, but it can still improve your LinkedIn profile.

IT'S ALL ABOUT NETWORKING TO IMPROVE YOUR CAREER

Many different groups on LinkedIn can help you connect with other professionals who share a common interest. Many of these users have questions for which you may have the answers. Being involved in LinkedIn groups can make you an influencer and help your profile get the attention of hiring managers.

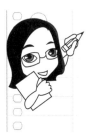

NERDY NOTE

A great way to get noticed by hiring managers and recruiters is to post helpful replies to discussions in LinkedIn groups. You are helping the community by giving your insight, and you are letting potential employers know that you are knowledge-able about the topic. It's a win-win!

LinkedIn allows users with free memberships a limited insight into who is visiting their profiles. If you opt to upgrade to a premium account, you can see all this information. However, even with the free account, you can get vital information regarding who is peeking at your profile. This is a helpful tool for you to determine which of your skill sets is drawing the attention of potential viewers. A good piece of advice is that if you notice hiring managers or recruiters looking at your profile, it is totally acceptable to send them connection invitations. This action lets them know that you are open to a conversation and interested in potentially expanding your career horizons.

Even if you aren't currently looking for a job, it is always a good idea to keep your resume fresh. LinkedIn is the new version of a resume, so you should take the time to make sure it is accurate and shows your strengths. You never know when a new opportunity will come your way, and you will want to be able to strike while the iron is hot.

GOOGLE+

Google+ is the baby of the major social networks. It is powered by the strength of Google and can be described as a combination of Twitter and Facebook but with the added benefit of actually influencing search rankings through its +1 feature. The social media platform is elegant in design and offers some great features; however, it is often overshadowed by Facebook's widespread use. Don't overlook this network, though, because it offers some really useful tools, such as communities, hangouts, and hashtags (#).

The +1 feature (and its related integrated website button) greatly improves overall search rankings if you include it in your posts. The +1 feature is similar to a like on Facebook because it is easy to click and is often incorporated onto other websites. This functions as a way of signifying that you like the content, you agree with the poster, or that you find the entry interesting. The Internet runs on popularity, and where you appear in Google search results can determine whether your business thrives or fails. Google+ gives you the ability to influence those search rankings by taking your +1 into consideration when determining those rankings.

Google+ works a little differently, because it lets you categorize different people into circles and then easily choose to share content with those specific circles. This simplicity is a breath of fresh air for people who are concerned with the frequently changing privacy settings of Facebook. With circles, you can separate your friends into defined groups that will better help you determine whom you share your status updates with. If you want to share an update with your nurse friends, just select the nurse group. If you want the entire world to see your update, then you can choose to make your status public. For example, you can have a group just for family members and share updates related to the birth of your child only with your family circle. Google+ makes this act a little easier by having you specify who can see your update while you are posting it, although Google+ automatically assumes that you want to share updates with the last group you shared with. This default can be helpful if you are constantly sharing with the same group of people. Many users find this transparency refreshing in a world of constantly changing standards.

CODE CAUTION

Make sure you pay attention to whom are you sharing updates with. If you only want to share with your family, you need to remember that the default sharing setting is going to be based upon your last update. This is easy to see when you are posting and can quickly be changed. Just make sure you are taking the time to ensure that you've selected the correct sharing circles.

Google+ communities are where you can connect to others who share a common interest. There are groups for nurses in general and nursing specialties. Much like other social networks, you can share links, images, and status updates. These are helpful resources to share thoughts and opinions with other nurses. If you ever need support or advice, communities are a great way to get them.

I use Google+ pretty regularly and am trying to increase my focus on this network. As a blogger, it's imperative that I use it because social interaction here can make a big difference in search engine rankings. The communities are also a great area to connect with others sharing a common interest. In my experience, the organization feels a little more global and less segregated than Facebook or even Twitter.

In reality, Google+ is probably a better social network than many of the others, but it's still a baby compared to the other key players. With time, I wouldn't be surprised if Google+ became the favorite social network and Facebook was laughed about like MySpace is today.

FORUMS

Forums are one of the best places to get focused attention on discussions. By design, forums cater to groups with common interests, and individualism is often sacrificed for the greater good of the group effort. Many nurse-centric online forums are well maintained and frequently visited by many nurses, who really appreciate the community they provide and their focus on a common theme.

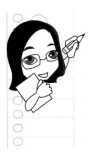

NERDY NOTE

Without a doubt, the most popular nursing forum is allnurses.com. However, Nurse-Together (www.nursetogether.com), NursingLink (http://nursinglink.monster.com), and the forums at Nurse.com (http://forums.nurse.com/) are all lively as well. Each forum offers a unique design and layout. Many nurses do prefer one forum over another for various reasons.

HOW FORUMS DIFFER FROM OTHER SOCIAL MEDIA PLATFORMS

One of the biggest differences between forums and Facebook or perhaps Twitter is how they appear in search engines. If you create a topic in a forum and it gets many responses, then Google will generally rank it higher. Facebook groups aren't indexed at all by Google, so if you want to find those results, you have to search Facebook directly.

Forums allow many to voice their opinions about a topic. Short of moderation for inappropriate content, forum content is typically left as it is received. Most forums do not rank forum replies, and therefore they appear in the order they are posted. This really helps promote the community aspect of forum posts, because one post or reply is not more important than another, with the exception of "sticky posts." Sticky posts are typically rules, guidelines, notices, or other announcements to forum users and therefore need to be seen first.

Forums do often sacrifice individuality for the greater goals of the group. Profiles are generally small, and many do not even bother filling them out. Some forums allow you to place links or quotes in your signature for personal self-expression, but the popular forum at allnurses.com does not. Although a signature is not a requirement of a good forum, many appreciate this feature and choose to use other forums when this option is not available.

I actually created a forum post asking about this policy on allnurses.com and was quickly told by a forum moderator that if I wanted to advertise, I should purchase advertising. This quick reaction really put a foul taste in my mouth and made me feel like it was more about money than community.

If you want to get focused attention on a topic, then nursing forums are an excellent avenue. With many other social networks, you might find that your post gets lost in the crowd. With a forum, the chances of it not being seen are drastically reduced, because the people coming to a forum for nurses are looking to talk about nursing specifically.

BLOGGING

Blogging is a way that many nurses can express their thoughts and opinions about the nursing profession and health care in general on their own terms. Many nurses turn to blogging when they feel the need to voice their opinions to a larger audience than their immediate social circle. They may also be interested in nursing entrepreneurship, expanding their writing ability, boosting their resumes, or connecting with other nurses. You can write about specific patient experiences as long as you keep HIPAA guidelines in mind and always respect the privacy of your patients and the social media policies of your employer.

SPEAKING TO THE WORLD

For me, blogging is a very personal thing. When I had my own personal struggles at work, I felt like I had already told everyone who would listen. I didn't want to burden my friends anymore with my frequent ramblings of my frustrations in the nursing world, but I felt like I still needed an outlet, so I went online and told the world.

When you feel frustrated or like no one really understands what you are going through, receiving comments that you are helping others with the same scenario can be very uplifting. Blogging can be an excellent form of therapy for a nurse who needs to vent professional or personal frustrations and for other nurses who want to see how others are dealing with the same difficult situations.

I also knew that I had a positive message to share with an audience. Nursing should be about building people up and improving lives. When we are at the bedside, we can only touch a few lives at a time, but if we take our message to the Web and blog about it, we can touch the world.

ENTREPRENEURSHIP

Blogging is an excellent way for nurses to go into business for themselves. Many nurse coaches use blogs as a way to advertise their services and support their bodies of work. Many nurse writers use blogging to build their portfolios and audiences. Others use blogging as a mechanism for revenue directly on their blog through ad sales, endorsements, and other means.

Many nurses are surprised to learn that you can use the Internet as a means to earn income. But many nurses are making a living online by using their nursing background and expertise.

Nurses can use the Web to go into business for themselves in so many ways. I know one nurse who creates nursing-related artwork and images that are made into T-shirts and coffee mugs. She receives a commission for each product that is sold. She started out earning only a little, but over the years it has replaced her full-time income.

Another nurse I know has a serious of ebooks that she has written on topics that appeal to nursing students and new nurses. She uses the Web and social media to promote her products, and her sales continue to increase. The more books she writes, the higher her income goes!

Many nurse coaches operate almost exclusively virtually. They create many different types of info-products ranging from mastermind courses to evaluation tools. These nurses thrive in their businesses, because they fill a need that others aren't.

The keys to being a successful nurse entrepreneur are patience, persistence, and passion. If you don't have a ton of these qualities, then move on over and let the next nurse step to the front of the line.

If you think you do have what it takes, then start exploring your options. Find something that you can be good at and see where it goes. You can get started for free and then grow a business slowly. Online businesses have little overhead and are flexible, and many nurses find the ability to be their own boss very appealing.

WRITING

Even though the narrative nursing note is quickly going the way of the dinosaur, a nurse should never be without good writing skills. Blogging can allow you to discuss nursing in ways that you cannot while delivering patient care. It can give you the opportunity to discuss your feelings and desires related to the nursing profession.

Nursing is difficult and yields many experiences that are worthy of writing down. Many nurses struggle from emotional disturbances and posttraumatic stress from their experiences, so writing can be a form of therapy. Putting these thoughts online in blog form can also help other nurses, who may be able to identify with you and your experiences.

According to Baikie and Wilhelm (2005), there are also many physical and emotional benefits of expressive writing, including:

✛ Reduced stress

✛ Reduced blood pressure

✛ Improved mood

✛ Improved memory

✛ Improved physical performance

You can also use writing to help you mold your career goals in nursing. You should take the time to write out where you visualize yourself to be in nursing in the coming years. Because writing goals down makes them more tangible, they therefore become more attainable. You can then review these goals later and be responsible for them. If you never write them down, you will be far less likely to review them with any real purpose of follow-through later.

Self-reflection is one of the best benefits of blogging. As nurses, we are so often consumed with caring for others that we forget to take time to care for ourselves. We need to take time every day to focus on our personal mental health and reflect on our experiences. Writing can help you think more deeply about things that interest you and get your ideas out on paper. It can also help free you of burdensome thoughts by relieving you from the stress of holding them in.

RESUME

You can use blogging and writing as a means to improve your resume. You can work as a free-lance writer, practice resume-writing skills, or even learn how to use content management system software. Each of these skills can boost your resume and help you achieve your career goals.

Many websites hire freelance writers on a per-article or hourly basis. All sorts of topics are available, and some of them even include health-related content. The pay for freelance writing can vary wildly, ranging from as little as a few dollars for an article to several hundred dollars for 500 words or so. As your writing improves and you gain recognition, your rates will rise.

Freelance writing is an excellent skill to put on your resume. Many administrative nursing roles require strong writing skills and creativity to get the job done—not to mention the extra income you can earn for putting words on the page.

CONNECTING

Blogging gives you the ability to connect with other nurses who are interested in the topics you are writing about. Right now you can Google just about any topic and find many related blogs that show up in your search results. If you visit those blogs, you often have the ability to comment on the entries and communicate directly with the author as well as other readers who have commented on the posts.

Blogs usually have social sharing icons embedded with the content (Figure 3.1). If you are reading a blog that you think is interesting and want to share it with your friends on Facebook or Twitter, you can usually do so easily by clicking on a share icon on the posts. Bloggers typically design their sites so that their articles can be shared as easily as possible, which usually makes a better viewing experience for the audience.

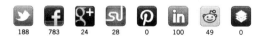

Figure 3.1 Social Media Shares Using Flare

Whether you choose to write your own blog or read and comment on others, you can benefit from the connections you can gain from blogs. Sharing your thoughts, ideas, knowledge, and expertise with the world is valuable for you and others. Don't be afraid to put yourself out there. You just might be pleasantly surprised.

BLOGGING AT THE NERDY NURSE

When I first started blogging, I had no idea where it was going to take me. It started as a personal outlet and a way to talk to the world. What I didn't anticipate is that the world would actually listen—and not only listen but talk back!

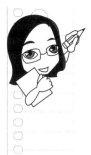

NERDY NOTE

If you happen to write a nursing blog, then no doubt the grammar and spelling police will be sure to let you know of any mistakes you've made. I've written several well-received articles that have had the grammar trolls out in full force. They have publicly (and sometimes anonymously) attacked my professionalism and my intelligence all over a misused word. I have learned from this experience to be cautious about what I publish, and I follow the Santa Claus method: Write a blog post and check it twice.

As I've gained an audience, blogging has become a bigger responsibility. What started as casual postings with little attention to detail have now become structured entries for which I pay great attention to detail, grammar, and search engine optimization (SEO). I had no idea how much work putting words on the Internet would be until after I got started and things started to grow.

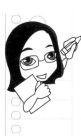

NERDY NOTE

SEO is important because it helps the cream rise to the top in search engine results. If someone is searching for an article about "nursing shoes" and you've written something really awesome about them, you want to make sure readers can find your post. The basic principles include inserting the main topic or keyword of your article in the title of your post, referring to this keyword again in the first paragraph, and linking to reliable and relevant content on this topic.

You can use tools like Google AdWords (http://adwords.google.com) to help you determine which keywords are most effective. If you want to get targeted traffic for a specific topic, you want to make sure you are using words that people are looking for. AdWords can give you an idea of the words people use when they search, how many people search for a topic, and how many people write about the topic. If at all possible, you want to choose keywords that don't have a lot of competition.

There's a whole lot of other nitty-gritty, deep-down nerdy stuff we could get into about SEO, but that's a topic for another day.

I spend at least an hour every weekday and more time on the weekends working on the blog and related social media areas. It has also created other opportunities online for me, such as freelance writing, being a brand ambassador for ScrubsMag.com, and going to conferences and events to speak on topics I've written about. I like to call conferences free vacations, but in reality, a lot of work and preparation goes into speaking at an event.

One of the most impressive outcomes I've had from blogging is landing a job as an informatics nurse. I was able to leverage the skills I learned while managing a database-driven content management system (Wordpress) on my resume and during my interview. I was apprehensive about putting my blog on my resume at first, because I know how fearful health care is of social media, but it was the best decision I ever made. I can now talk freely and openly about my blog, and it has also made me more much accountable for the content I create.

TECH TIP

It's one thing to have experience with technology; it's quite another to know how to fix it when it breaks. Although you won't learn how to do everything at once, if you run into technical issues, you should try to learn to fix them on your own.

Google is your friend here! If you don't know the answer, Google it!

I typically write posts one or two days a week and schedule them in advance. This is helpful when I'm working on other projects, because I can manage my time a little more efficiently. I also automate as much of the process as possible through Wordpress plug-ins. These automatically share my posts on Twitter and Facebook once they are published and help with SEO.

I often get compliments on "The Nerdy Nurse" name and branding, and people ask me how I came up with it. Because I was writing about things I experienced as a nurse, I knew I wanted "nurse" in the title, but I didn't want to be segregated into one niche. I also wanted to write about technology, do product reviews, and cover other lifestyle topics. Because my friends were always calling me a "nerd" (and I thought this was funny), The Nerdy Nurse was born.

HIPAA AND SOCIAL MEDIA POLICIES

If you choose to write about your experiences delivering patient care, you should always respect the privacy of your patients and their families. It is best that you avoid discussing any scenario that is extremely rare or could be pinpointed based upon your geographic location and time.

You should also make sure that you are aware of your employer's social media policy.

HIPAA defines 18 patient identifiers as off-limits:

1. Names

2. All geographical subdivisions smaller than a state, including street address, city, county, precinct, zip code, and their equivalent geocodes, except for the initial three digits of a zip code, if according to the current publicly available data from the Bureau of the Census: (1) The geographic unit formed by combining all zip codes with the same three initial digits contains more than 20,000 people; and (2) the initial three digits of a zip code for all such geographic units containing 20,000 or fewer people is changed to 000

3. All elements of dates (except year) for dates directly related to an individual, including birth date, admission date, discharge date, date of death; and all ages over 89 and all elements of dates (including year) indicative of such age, except that such ages and elements may be aggregated into a single category of age 90 or older

4. Phone numbers

5. Fax numbers

6. Electronic mail addresses

7. Social Security numbers

8. Medical record numbers

9. Health plan beneficiary numbers

10. Account numbers

11. Certificate/license numbers

12. Vehicle identifiers and serial numbers, including license plate numbers

13. Device identifiers and serial numbers

14. Web Universal Resource Locators (URLs)

15. Internet Protocol (IP) address numbers

16. Biometric identifiers, including finger- and voice prints

17. Full-face photographic images and any comparable images

18. Any other unique identifying number, characteristic, or code (note that this does not mean the unique code assigned by the investigator to code the data)

Note: You can find a one-page document formatted and ready for printing off this information at www.TheNerdyNurse.com/HIPAA.

(Original source: UC Berkeley Research Administration and Compliance, n.d.).

Patients put a great deal of trust in their nurses, and they deserve to have their privacy maintained. It is important that you ensure that patients or their families cannot be identified by any online writing you produce. If you choose to blog about the care you deliver, your focus should be about your experiences and not about specific patients. Most nurse bloggers scramble their patients into combined versions and have explicit disclosures stating this fact.

If you choose to blog openly with your name and profession attached to your blog, you should know that your readers will likely determine your geographic location. If there is a particularly rare phenomenon that occurs at your medical facility and you take part in the affected patient's care, it is probably best that you refrain from writing about said event.

An anesthesiologist crossed some major ethical lines when she chose to tweet about a priapism she was called in to assist with at 4 a.m. Because a priapism isn't your average everyday medical ailment and the health care provider's location could be easily determined, many believed that the author of said tweet revealed too much. Think seriously about what you write, and if you feel it may be close to crossing the HIPAA line, do not write it. You should also take the time to get familiar with your employer's social media policy. Whether you are blogging or just posting status updates on Facebook, make sure that you fall within the guidelines your employer has established when you participate in online activity.

HOW HOSPITALS SHOULD USE SOCIAL MEDIA

If your health care organization's administrators have not already created a social media policy, they need to step up to the plate and get with the program. Patients are looking for you online before, during, and after their visits. Social media has given them a voice, and they use it frequently. But a health care organization's staff members have been given this very same voice, and they can use this voice to enhance the lives of the patients they serve.

It is imperative that a health care organization's leadership not be afraid of social media. Are hospital staff members afraid of the patients they care for? I certainly hope not. Social media is about engaging and connecting with patients, professionals, and others who are involved in all the workings of health care.

If your health care organization does not already have an official blog, a staff member needs to be appointed to start one. These are valuable resources for patients and employees that can be used to share important information about the health care organization or pertinent health topics. Social media in health care is a way to educate and provide resources to the communities that hospitals serve.

If a patient has questions about a procedure, a physician, or your renovation, a blog and other forms of social media can help provide the information in a transparent way that promotes trust. Transparency and authenticity are so vital in health care. If you aren't talking about the great things you are doing in health care, then people might assume you aren't doing anything. My mother once told me, "If you don't toot your own horn, no one is going to know that it blows." Use social media to toot your horn and respond to the community that you serve.

SOCIAL MEDIA AS A STAFF NURSE

As a staff nurse, your utilization of social media will be very different. Unless your role includes social media, it is probably wise if you refrain from listing your employer in your social media profiles. The reasons for this are simple: If you identify yourself as an employee, then you label yourself as a representative of your organization in that medium. Sometimes people say things on Facebook and Twitter that would not reflect well upon their employers. So unless you can ensure that you'll be 100% professional 100% of the time, it is best that you not involve your employer in your social media activities.

That is not to say, however, that you cannot own your nursing expertise online.

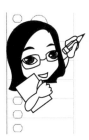

NERDY NOTE
As The Nerdy Nurse, I own every bit of my nursing and expertise online; I am just not acting as a representative of the health care system that employs me. Its administrators are aware and supportive of my online activities, but we agree that I do not speak on their behalf.

So before you type in *Prestigious Memorial Medical Center, ICU, 3rd Floor* on that Facebook profile of yours, think long and hard about whether every statement you make online would represent your employer in the light in which it wishes to be represented. Freedom of speech is alive and well, and we should all embrace it, but not at the risk of embarrassing ourselves or our employers because we filled in more blanks on our profile than we probably should have.

FRIENDING YOUR PATIENTS ON FACEBOOK

Much controversy exists over the topic of whether you should friend your patients on Facebook. We care for our patients, and we are friendly toward them, but there are lines that should be drawn in the nurse-patient relationship. In an era where the lines between friends and mere acquaintances are often blurred, it can be difficult to know which decision to make when a patient you have cared for extends a friend request.

In nursing, we start our care anticipating a discharge and planning for that moment from day one. We have to ensure that even though we greatly enjoy our patients and being able to care for them, we cannot allow ourselves to become invested in them outside the health care role. There are exceptions to this guideline, of course, and you can use your own personal judgment to determine when this is the case. But as a rule, it's probably not a good idea to encourage Ms. Perfect Patient to friend you on Facebook after one shift of caring for her.

"Why not?" you ask. Well, allow me to present just one scenario that you probably haven't considered.

During college, you may have "partied it up" with the best of them. The memories you have from those days are hazy at best, and you're glad that Facebook wasn't around back then to haunt you. But do you remember those keg stands you did 20 years ago? Yes, *those* keg stands. Someone snapped photos of those potentially regrettable events and has posted them on Facebook. And if that weren't bad enough, this person has added insult to injury by tagging you in every one of them. When those pictures appear on Facebook and on your wall, Ms. Perfect Patient isn't too impressed with your behavior.

You can use your imagination to fill in the rest of this story. It could potentially end with her calling hospital administrators and discussing how she believes that your behavior is unbecoming of a respectable nurse. It could lead to an awkward conversation in the director of nursing's office. Or you could avoid the situation altogether by not friending your patient on Facebook.

Now technically, Ms. Perfect Patient could still decide to find you on Facebook on her own, but if you're smart and you have your account's security settings chosen appropriately, she won't be able to see those keg stand pictures without first requesting to be your friend.

TECH TIP

Setting up your Facebook privacy settings is easy:

+ After you've logged into Facebook, click on the gear/cog on the upper right side. Then click "Privacy Settings."

+ Edit "Who can see my stuff" and "Who can look me up" to a setting that feels comfortable.

+ Pat yourself on the back. You've secured your profile!

Every day in nursing, we have to critically think to provide the best patient care. I urge you to do some intense critical thinking about how you choose to use social media in relationship to your nursing career.

WRAPPING IT UP

Oh my goodness. This was a busy chapter, wasn't it? Are you swimming in social media yet? Have you started a Twitter account? Did you clean up your privacy settings on Facebook?

Here are a couple of questions that you should be able to answer now:

+ What is a hashtag?

+ Why is Google+ important to website owners and bloggers?

+ How can you impress hiring managers and recruiters on LinkedIn?

REFERENCES

Baikie, K. A., & Wilhelm, K. (2005). Emotional and physical health benefits of expressive writing. *Advances in Psychiatric Treatment, 11,* 338–346. Retrieved from http://apt.rcpsych.org/content/11/5/338.full

UC Berkeley Research Administration and Compliance. (n.d.). HIPAA PHI: List of 18 identifiers and definition of PHI. Retrieved from http://cphs.berkeley.edu/hipaa/hipaa18.html

4

GETTING EXCITED ABOUT COMPUTERS

Computers are modern marvels and incredible pieces of machinery. We often forget to acknowledge how amazing all their masterful capabilities truly are. Rather, we get bogged down on their current complications and inconveniences, because our attention is always on the latest and greatest design that is lighter and thinner than the current model. What we have to remember is how far computers have come. The general rule is that the longer we have a certain technology, the more user-friendly it becomes. Like all technology, computers are forever changing, and one area of life they continue to improve is delivery of nursing care.

Computers are so ubiquitous in our lives today that we probably couldn't imagine life without them—from grocery store checkout lanes to the smartphone (or even not-so-smartphones) you use every day. Do you have a GPS in your car? Have you programmed your DVR lately? Have you documented patient medical records at work? Just take a moment to think of anything electronic you use—chances are these items probably contain computers.

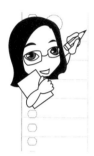

NERDY NOTE

Do you use a glucose meter or electronic vital signs machine to care for your patients? There are computers in those too!

If you work for a really tech-savvy employer, the results you get from these may even be streamed wirelessly and automatically update the patients' electronic medical records (EMRs).

Gone are the days when parents gave their kids Legos to keep their minds busy or sent them outside to play in the yard and blow off some energy. Now parents use tablets and DVRs to keep kids occupied. With the advent of learning technology and websites for kids, sometimes you may feel like the average 3-year-old knows more about computers than you do.

Because of the intuitiveness of many smartphones, tablets, and touch-screen computers, children often have an easier time using computers than adults. But that doesn't mean that anyone with an interest should have any real trouble learning to use a computer effectively. And besides, are you really going to let the kids have all the fun?

USING A COMPUTER TO IMPROVE NURSING CARE

With the Meaningful Use mandate going full force, most health care organizations have adopted electronic documentation systems. This means that as a nurse, you will be expected to use a computer to document your nursing care. Many nurses loathe documenting in an EMR and believe that paper charting is much more efficient. But I'll let you in on a little secret: It's not.

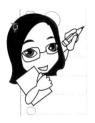

NERDY NOTE
Think about all the new requirements that nurses now are required to document. Can you even imagine trying to do all *that* on paper?

Using an EMR may feel cumbersome and inconvenient, but it's likely because you are apprehensive about using the system. EMR systems give you quick access to all the information you need to care for your patients, more insight into their histories, and a more well-rounded look at their overall conditions. As nurses, we strive to practice holistic care and treat the person, not just the disease. Having full access to a patient's health information can help us gain a greater understanding of what that person's "normal" is and help us determine what we need to do to get the patient back to that point.

Using a computer also ensures that documentation for patients is completely legible. This means that orders are clear and notes related to patient care are easily read and understood. Eventually the skill of deciphering physician handwriting will no longer be needed. If orders are entered electronically, there is no guesswork involved in interpreting what the order says and overall fewer errors occur.

CONNECTING WITH YOUR NURSING TRIBE

Countless nurses online are looking to communicate with other nurses. New nurses are looking for seasoned mentors. Experienced nurses are seeking a new outlook on their careers. Satisfied (or unsatisfied) nurses simply want an opportunity to express themselves.

Although you may be fortunate to have friends outside work who are also nurses and therefore understand the unique jobs you do, you may still want to connect with others and become a part of a bigger group. Computers can give you more opportunities for connection and belonging than you could ever hope to find offline. What makes online communities even more useful is the fact that you can find nurses with similar backgrounds to yours who can act as excellent sounding boards when you have questions and concerns or feel burned-out.

As we discussed in Chapter 3, there are a variety of ways to connect with other nurses online. My personal favorite is through nursing blogs—websites that are written by a nurse, or group of nurses, that discuss topics related to patient care, nursing issues, and general subjects related to the nursing lifestyle. Nurses in all types of specialties write blogs. Many of these bloggers are writing from their hearts, are not endorsed by a business or company, and are unpaid for their time to write. They offer personal insight into the world of nursing and can be an excellent resource if you are looking for a connection that you may not have been able to find in your workplace.

As a nurse blogger myself, I am a little biased toward the blogging platform, but I believe it offers the best opportunity for personal and professional growth for nurses online. Commenting and interacting with a blog's author and readers can give you personal satisfaction and possibly even the opportunity to leave a lasting impression on articles that nurses may read for many years to come. Blogging is all about having a conversation and being involved in a community, and it takes people to make that happen. Even if you did not create the original blog post, your words can still make a difference to others.

Blogging can be therapeutic. It can give you the opportunity to explore topics that interest you and allow you to write about them in a conversational style that is vastly different than any of the formal writing you ever did in nursing school. Nurse bloggers have the unique opportunity to influence the nursing community without going through a professional organization or having a large amount of money to forward an agenda. They can reach nurses one-on-one and promote positive changes in health care. If you have a message that you believe needs to be shared, then blogging can get you connected to your tribe and allow you to spread that message throughout the world. It is worth noting that if you can imagine it, then someone's probably written a blog about it, and if no one else has, then you should start one yourself.

You're probably already using a computer at home but may not know as much about it as you'd like. In this chapter, I talk a little about good habits when purchasing a computer, how to set up and maintain your computer, password management, and mobile computing solutions. I also share some tips and tricks to save you time and effort when using a computer that might even be able to save you time while documenting in an EMR. I also discuss some new computer technology that is available for TVs.

Ensure that your posterior is firmly planted in a chair, because you're not going to want to miss this one.

BUYING A COMPUTER

Buying a computer for personal use can be a bit overwhelming. Take it from me—I've bought a nearly a dozen in my life, and each one has been a difficult purchase to make. My suggestion for computer buyers is to go to a retail store that specializes in electronics. Hardly any of their employees work on commission anymore, so you don't need to be afraid that they are just going to try and sell you something because it is more expensive. Consumer electronics associates are trained to assess your needs for a computer and point you in the direction of one that will best meet them. If you are a first-time buyer, you might find that they are asking you many questions.

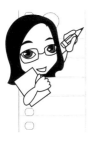

NERDY NOTE

Although it's recommended that you go to a store that specializes in electronics to look at computers, you don't necessarily have to buy them there. If you want to save a little extra money, many online retailers do not charge sales tax and will ship your desired system to your door for free.

Typical questions might include the following:

+ What do you plan on doing with your computer?

+ Would you like your computer to be portable? Do you travel?

+ Do you plan to edit and share photos online?

+ Do you listen to a lot of music? Do you use iTunes, Pandora, or Spotify?

+ Do you want to interact with family and friends via social media?

+ Do you have a preference for an operating system, such as Windows versus Mac?

+ Do you want to get rid of your regular television set and just watch TV or movies online?

+ Do you want to use Skype or another video application to talk with family and friends?

+ Are you trying to save money by consolidating your phone, television, and Internet services via a computer?

+ Do you want to use your computer to control your home entertainment systems and stream your videos on your TV?

+ Do you have a husband, son, or daughter (or you!) who is an avid online gamer?

Your employer likely has several different types of computers that you use to document your nursing care. You should be well versed in how to interact with any computer you encounter. This adaptability is a skill that employers value, and it will reduce your overall stress level when you're learning new things. The good news is that whether the computer is a laptop, desktop, or tablet, it shouldn't take much time to get acquainted with a new piece of technology. It's kind of like riding a bike—once you know how, getting on a new one is just a matter of feeling it out and then going for a ride.

No one computer is better suited for nurses to own over others, but laptops definitely have an advantage. Tablets are also extremely portable and often used in places where a laptop wouldn't be. If you're reading up on research concerning a particular nursing issue, then a tablet can be handy to access this information while you are on the go.

TECH TIP

If you want to use a tablet but hate typing on the touch screen, there is a solution for you! Many cases have small keyboards incorporated into them, which are usually much easier to type on and can really help increase your productivity with a tablet.

Determining your primary usage for your computer will dictate what you need to purchase. To start, you need to look at basic memory and storage. You don't need to know all about it, but as you're deciphering the numbers in the advertising flyer, look first at memory and storage. Memory (RAM) determines how fast your machine will process or run. If you just need a machine at home to do papers, edit pictures, or stream video or social media, a minimum of 4GB in memory should be fine for you. But if you are an avid online gamer or need more processing capability to edit live video files, then look for something with a bit more power.

Next, look at storage capacity. Hard drives are measured in MB or GB. Every 1GB (gigabyte) equals 1,000MB (megabytes). A 200GB hard drive may sound huge, but if you plan to keep thousands of photos and your entire 600-album R&B collection on your hard drive, it won't be nearly large enough.

If you're buying a desktop computer, you may get a choice of monitors. You'll need to decide which size and quality work for you. Most people won't notice a difference in refresh rate or resolution, but if you are editing images or videos you might.

If you decide to buy a laptop, you might notice that some of the newer models do not come with DVD/CD drives. This might seem shocking at first, but there is a very good reason why they are no longer being included: People don't use them, and they take up a lot of space. Most would rather have a thinner, lighter laptop, so the disc drive is sacrificed.

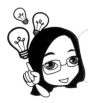

TECH TIP

If you think you might need or want a disc drive for a computer that doesn't have one, you can purchase a separate external drive for around $50.

Do you have a printer at home already? Do you know whether it will be compatible? Is the ink expensive? Should you upgrade to a new model? Printing technology has improved at the same rate as computers. Some printers can do almost everything for you except cook your breakfast with their scanning, faxing, and photo-printing capabilities. The newer ink is usually much more affordable and easier to find than the old toners.

TECH TIP

USB ports are the ubiquitous connection ports for everything from your wireless mouse to your network printer. Most computers come with two to six built in, but what if you have every port filled before you plug in your iPod and a portable flash drive? Look for a USB expansion port, which takes up one plug on the computer but—sort of like a power strip—gives you another eight to work with.

WHERE TO BUY

Have you given any thought to where you will purchase a computer? Many people like to touch and interact with a computer before they take it home. This convenience may end up costing you money, however, because if you buy a computer in a brick-and-mortar location, you are going to have to pay sales tax and be pestered to buy extra add-ons, even though most retailers no longer pay sales associates on commission.

Buying a computer online can be a much more enjoyable experience than going to the store because you are in control of what you look at and what you think is important. It's also sweet to save all that extra money on tax, especially because websites like Newegg.com and Amazon.com usually offer free shipping as well.

EXTENDED WARRANTY: GO OR NO?

I worked at Circuit City when I was in nursing school and sold my fair share of extended warranties. I can tell you firsthand that even though most consumer electronics retailers do not pay their employees commission, these sales associates are pressured to achieve a certain percentage of extended warranty sales. If you ever feel like you're being pressured into buying a warranty, this is probably why.

But a warranty shouldn't be completely avoided. On major electronic purchases, such as computers, tablets, and televisions, an extended warranty can help stretch the life of your product. A general rule of thumb is to spend 10% or less of the price of the product on the warranty.

NERDY NOTE

You consider the expectation for the life of the product before buying a warranty, right? If you plan to own a computer for several years before replacing it, then an extended warranty, if priced affordably, is a worthwhile investment.

One of the best pieces of advice I can give you is to know whether you want the warranty before the sales pitch begins. Whether you buy your computer in a store or online, there's going to be a push for the warranty. The salesperson is going to mention it at every available opportunity. Some web pages will have the offer pop up multiple times before you can complete the sale. If you aren't careful, you may accidently buy it. However, if you've made the decision beforehand, you will have no trouble completing the sale.

CREDIT CARD PROTECTION AND INCENTIVES

Some credit card companies, including American Express and Platinum Visa, actually double the warranty for electronics that you buy. You need to check with your card issuer to determine the terms of the warranty and how to make sure you qualify. Most require you to register your device through their service within the standard warranty's time frame.

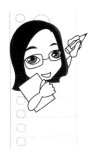

NERDY NOTE

Most manufacturers' warranties cover 1 year of parts and labor for internal components on your device. This does not usually include software you've installed on the machine or removal of malware (spyware and viruses). However, even if the company states that it doesn't support software, most provide basic troubleshooting or fixes for issues that you encounter related to the computer's operating system.

You may also be offered special financing on certain store credit cards. This can be helpful for large purchases, because you can spread your payments out over time. You may have the ability to earn rewards points on the same credit card for making the purchase at a particular location.

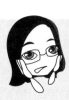

CODE CAUTION

Make sure you are aware of the terms of the credit card you are using when it comes to no interest/no payments for a specific amount of time. If you buy something on 12 months same-as-cash, you typically have to pay off the balance in full within 12 months to avoid being slapped with every bit of the interest you would have accrued during that time.

SETTING UP AND FIXING UP

If you have bought a new computer, then the setup is fairly straightforward. You might be asked a few questions about your location, your wireless network password, and maybe your email address. If you buy your computer in a brick-and-mortar store, an employee may complete these steps for you, but there is really no need for someone else to do it. If you can follow directions, the computer's startup wizard will guide you through the process.

Most computers come with a trial of antivirus software, which helps ensure that you are protected from malware threats while surfing the Internet. Many different companies produce this software, including McAfee and Symantec, but most technology experts agree that any of them will get the job done. If your computer comes with a free trial, you might as well take advantage of it. After the trial runs out, you will need to pay an annual subscription fee to continue coverage.

I'm probably setting myself up to be jinxed here, but I don't usually run additional antivirus software. Windows computers come with Windows defender free and a built-in firewall. I'm pretty aware of the websites I surf to, and I don't click on anything questionable, open any email I am unsure of, or download any files that I don't know the origin of. This practice has served me well so far and complements my frugal nature.

TECH TIP

I do recommend antivirus software for the average technology consumer. I just like to live dangerously, and I'm really, *really* cheap.

If you run into problems with your computer, your first resource should be the manufacturer. Look in your paperwork or do a quick Google search to find the manufacturer's support contact information. If the problem occurs within 12 months of purchase, most manufacturers will help you correct problems over the phone or have you send the computer in for service if it requires parts to be exchanged. In this situation, most computer manufacturers provide prepaid shipping labels, so there is no out-of-pocket cost.

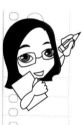

NERDY NOTE

It's important that you keep certain items when you buy a computer. You should keep your original box and packaging for 30 days. If you notice any problems within the first 30 days, you should return the computer directly to the store. Most stores will not accept returns for technology items without the original box, related cables, paperwork, and a copy of the receipt.

You should store copies of your receipt and any barcodes with serial numbers. I recommend doing this digitally by using a smartphone app to take a picture of the label and then store the image on a cloud-based server, like Google Drive. You can also locate your serial numbers on the bottom of your computer.

Many people fill their basements with the boxes from every computer they've ever owned, but you don't actually have to do this. Most manufacturers will ship you a box to return your broken product for repairs free of charge. Those that don't ship a box often have arrangements with FedEx or UPS stores to package and ship your device on their dime.

So take a deep breath, say a few last parting words, and throw those old boxes away!

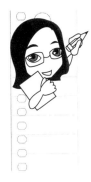

NERDY NOTE

What should you expect when you need help? Many computer repair experts can accurately diagnose and fix a problem without ever meeting you in person. When you call a computer or software company to figure out an issue, be prepared for the person helping you to access your machine remotely—but you need to make sure you only give this information to authorized support representatives from the computer manufacturer or other repair personnel whom you trust.

If you encounter a problem with your computer after your warranty has expired, you can attempt to troubleshoot the problem yourself by doing some Google searches. If the problem is more than you can handle, you should locate a reputable computer repair store or trusted family member or friend to do the repairs. If you have a friend who can do it, I'd probably go with this person, but it may not get fixed as quickly as if you took it to a legitimate computer repair store. However, if your friend's price is "free" or cheap, it might be worth the wait, because computer repairs can be costly.

CODE CAUTION

One of the reasons I became technologically inclined is because I'm frugal. I didn't want to pay others to fix things that I was sure I could do myself. It turns out that I was right, and I can fix most things myself. Some computer repair stores take advantage of people who don't know very much about computers. Be aware of this, and don't let anyone swindle you.

PASSWORD, PASSWORD, WHO'S GOT THE PASSWORD?

If I have one password, I swear I have 100. It's so hard to keep track of the different user logins that I use for the business, blogging, and banking. Each website has a different set of password requirements, and nearly every password expert on the planet recommends that you don't use the same one over and over again.

CODE CAUTION

The reason you shouldn't use the same password over and over again is pretty straight-forward: If hackers get the password to one of your accounts, they then have it for all your accounts.

So how do you keep up with the hundreds of user names and passwords that you are expected to remember? A few really good apps help you manage your passwords and user names securely and even help you back them up online. My personal favorite is RoboForm, but I've also had experience with LastPass. In general, LastPass didn't feel as powerful to me, but admittedly, I was already using RoboForm and was probably expecting it do things it wasn't designed to do. What can I say, though—I'm a tough nerd to please.

I started using RoboForm back in my pro-sweeper days and really liked the fact that I could save all my information in one location, including addresses, passwords, and even security questions. It also has a mobile app available so that you can use it while on the go.

CODE CAUTION

One quirk about RoboForm is that even though you can access stored data and fill in passwords on the mobile app, you cannot save new passwords to the mobile app. Because of this, it's not a good solution for any of your nursing and work passwords.

1Password, LastPass, and mSecure are password-management solutions that offer the ability to store passwords via smartphone apps as well as sync them to desktop applications. They enable you to securely store your information with one master password, which can help ease the headache of remembering so many different passwords by letting you conveniently store them in one secure location.

SIMPLIFYING COMPUTER USE

You may already be using a computer at home, but you might not know about some of the useful shortcuts and tricks that are available to you.

Learning some basic keyboard shortcuts can be helpful in electronic documentation and general computer use. For example, pressing combinations of certain keys lets you complete basic word-processing functions.

Here are some of the most commonly used combinations:

ctrl + c = Copy
ctrl + v = Paste
ctrl + x = Cut
ctrl + a = Select All
ctrl + f = Find

Note: for Mac users, substitute the Command key for control.

These can be helpful in basic word processing or when using EMR systems that allow their use.

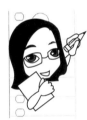

NERDY NOTE
The "find" feature can be used in many word-processing applications, PDF files, and most websites.

Another cool computer trick that I like to share with people is how to create a screen shot. If you are using Windows 7 or newer, you can use the handy-dandy snipping tool.

1. I recommend you find this tool under accessories in Windows 7 or through an app search in Windows 8.

2. Once you find the snipping tool, you can pin to your toolbar so that it's always handy.

3. After you have it available, just click on it, and it will turn your screen white; drag to select the area of the screen you want to capture.

4. You can then paste it into a document or save the image to your files.

Simple tricks like these can really make using your computer a much better experience and help you get things done so much faster. I find that many nurses are much happier computer users when they have shortcuts like this under their belt.

TECH TIP

If you don't have a snipping tool available, you can also do a print screen by simply clicking the button that says "PrtScn" located on the upper right side of your keyboard. This copies an image of everything that's on your screen to your clipboard, and you can then paste the image into a document or email. You can also crop the image to include only relevant details.

USING YOUR COMPUTER FOR NURSING

Most nurses have one primary consideration when it comes to determining which type of computer is right for them. For many it's budget, for some it's size, and for a growing number it's portability. You should also consider how you might want to use your computer to enhance your nursing practice.

Many health care organizations have policies against bringing personal laptops to work; however, most are lenient toward tablets and eReaders. Depending of the flow of your shift and the policies of your employer, you may be permitted to have a tablet at work. For many nurses, having tablets on their shift can be very helpful, giving them increased access to information and allowing them to stay connected.

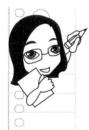

NERDY NOTE

Although many people have replaced their eReaders with fancier new tablets, old-school eReaders will always hold a special place in my heart. They helped pave the way for tablet technology and showed consumer electronics manufacturers and book creators that we don't need paper to enjoy a good book.

Nursing education, including formal schooling, is one of the key areas where you can use your computer for nursing. Although employers are sometimes at odds with the use of personal electronic devices, they sometimes make exceptions if you are pursuing higher nursing education or attempting to gain continuing education (CE) credits. In many states, you cannot practice without acquiring CE credits annually, and most employers are more than happy to let you earn those credits in your spare time while you are on the floor. Many online options are available for you to gain education credits on a free or paid basis. Having a tablet or computer handy can help you fulfill your requirements more quickly and reduce your overall stress level.

If you plan to purchase a single device to use, then you need to make sure it works the way you want it to. For example, most tablets have onscreen keyboards, but many skilled typists find them less than desirable for composing text documents. However, if your primary interest is reading, watching media, or surfing the Web, then a tablet would work fine for you.

In general terms, a traditional computer or laptop works much better for input tasks, such as composing a paper on a nursing theorist, creating any sort of content or media, editing images, and completing any other task that produces a file. If you want to produce something yourself, traditional computers tend to work best.

On the other hand, tablets work well for more passive tasks involving viewing, reading, or watching. This type of computer is great for reading nursing articles or watching videos related to a new procedure you are interested in learning about. Many people find that viewing content with a tablet is easier and more user-friendly than using a computer with a mouse and keyboard input. The intuitive nature of the touch entry tends to simplify the process and reduce complications.

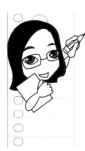

NERDY NOTE

Do you like to draw? Most tablets have some really cool drawing applications that can be used with your finger or, if you're feeling devoted, via a stylus that can be picked up for less than $20. Even if you're not an artist, it's fun to play around with these. Oh, and kids *love* using a stylus on tablets, which has the added benefit of keeping potentially grubby fingers off your screen.

Many find that they want more than one device to fulfill different functions, and if this is in your budget, having additional choices can be really nice. You can use your tablet to read an article while you use your computer to write about it or interact with friends on Facebook. These tasks can also be done on a single device, but some like the opportunity to have a different screen devoted to each task. Personally, I usually have three devices with me whenever I am within the range of Wi-Fi—my laptop, an iPad, and an iPhone. I use them all for different purposes and feel practically naked when I'm missing even one of them.

Choosing between a laptop and desktop is a matter of personal preference. The benefits of a laptop usually outweigh any detriments. The primary selling factor is its portability. Having a laptop can allow you to take your computer multiple places, whether it's an MSN class, the park, a restaurant, or just your front porch. It'd be pretty entertaining to watch you try to do all that with a desktop computer.

Many computers these days offer touch-screen experience, thus combining many aspects of a tablet with a computer. It is worth nothing that adding touch-screen capabilities to a laptop typically boosts the price by $200 to $300, and you can purchase a separate decent tablet, like the Kindle Fire, for the same price.

CODE CAUTION

If you use a tablet often, it is probably covered in germs. This becomes an even bigger issue if you are bringing your tablet to work or using a tablet at the bedside or in the field.

ZAGG.com offers ZAGGwipes and ZAGGfoam, which can be used to disinfect your electronic devices and zap bacteria on contact.

Tablets work best for shift nursing. If it's small enough, you can stick it in your pocket and carry it with you while you work. When you have a few minutes, you can read a few pages of a book or pursue other activities you enjoy. If you happen to work on a night shift and are lucky enough to have free time at work, buy a tablet. You'll thank me for it, I promise.

DOCUMENTING ELECTRONICALLY: ALL THE COOL KIDS ARE DOING IT

Many health care facilities are using electronic documentation to improve patient care and be compliant with Meaningful Use. Many facilities have taken a variety of approaches to making this happen, some of which work better than others.

As I referenced earlier, tablets work well for consumption but typically do not perform as well for input. In nursing, you input information when you document on an assessment, compose a narrative nursing note, or administer a medication. Because these actions require more than a few taps to the screen and the use of a keyboard, a tablet doesn't work as well. You can use laptop computers that have touch screens, which work a little better, but then you also have potential infection control issues, because these devices move from room to room.

Many hospitals use portable workstations. Depending on your facility, they may be called COWS (computers on wheels) or WOWS (workstations on wheels). They usually include a laptop or small desktop computer mounted to a rolling cart with a built-in internal battery. This option has the potential to be a good solution for bedside documentation but does have some downfalls.

WOWS usually have drawers and a work area that many nurses find helpful. You can often have a desk assigned to a single nurse and may even be able to lock items inside. This might be helpful to keep any paperwork you want to keep with you or saline flushes. However, they are usually large and heavy and can be cumbersome to carry from room to room. There is also the huge risk for infection-control issues because you will likely be rolling these carts in and out of patients' rooms. Even the best nurse can't keep up with sanitizing a cart completely in between patients, and it's best to avoid moving any object from room to room. Another concern is that the batteries in these degrade fairly quickly, and even though they may have lasted a full 12-hour shift the first year, a couple years down the road they might only last 30 minutes or an hour. Having to constantly plug in the WOWS to recharge between duties can be a challenge for many, especially if outlets are at a premium.

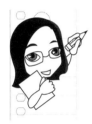

NERDY NOTE

Be sure to plug in WOWs so that they are fully charged for the next nurse that needs to use them. There is nothing worse than finding a mobile workstation only to discover that the battery is dead!

Many facilities opt to install desktop computers at the bedside. These are either mounted on the wall or stored in a compact cabinet. This solution tends to work better than WOWs, because nurses know there will always be a computer in the room, and they won't have to waste time chasing equipment. It also eliminates the infection-control issue related to any portable computer option.

CODE CAUTION

Check with your hospital administrators to make sure that computer equipment that remains in patient rooms is being cleaned between patients. This is a big issue that is often overlooked but can really be a huge source of germs. Keyboards should have covers that can be cleaned with Sani-Wipes, and computer mice should be wiped down as well.

If you find that you are using a device that does not work well for your electronic documentation needs, make time to discuss the concern with your manager. If management thinks that you are coping with what has been distributed, they are less likely to make changes when they are looking to order new equipment. You should know that the standard for replacing computers in health care is every 3 years. If your organization has had its equipment for a longer period of time, this can negatively affect your work performance due to slowness and other problems associated with outdated computer equipment.

It's up to you to be an advocate for what you need to take care of your patients. Electronic documentation can really help improve the nursing care you deliver, but not if you are using subpar equipment. Make sure you are advocating for what you need to deliver the best patient care possible and what will make your job not only easier but more productive.

TABLETS ARE WHERE IT'S AT

Many are finding that you rarely have to use a traditional computer anymore. A tablet or perhaps even a smartphone can fulfill most needs. You can do banking, social networking, messaging, web surfing, media viewing, gaming, and so much more on a tablet. The one area that you might find lacking is the touch-screen keyboard. However, most tablets allow you to sync a Bluetooth keyboard, and then you should be able to actually do some productive word processing.

However, as a frequent tablet user, I do find there are limitations to what can be done efficiently. Tablets in general work very well as consumption devices. If you want to look at it, read it, stream it, like it, or retweet it, then a tablet is the best choice. However, if you find yourself wanting to compose long messages or exchange emails longer than a few words, a tablet can become a bit frustrating. For me, I attribute this to the fact that I am a fairly fast typist when I have a good tangible keyboard to use. I just can't get over not feeling the punch and click of the keys on the tablet—that and the darn thing is always autocorrecting you, but that's a topic for another book.

If you are a hunt-and-peck typist, then a tablet will probably suit you just fine. A tablet is also beneficial for reading and viewing. Many enjoy browsing popular sites like Pinterest and StumbleUpon by using a tablet. There is little need for typing when browsing these websites, and they offer apps specifically designed for tablet use that make navigating these sites a breeze. If you wish to avoid using a full-fledged computer in most scenarios, a tablet can definitely get you connected and keep you mobile.

A tablet can be taken with you to work or play. If you're working on the floor, you can take a tablet with you to catch up on nursing articles and research while you have downtime at work. If you are pursuing higher nursing education, you can also access your online classroom via tablet and work on school projects in places other than your home.

Another way tablets can help you in your nursing practice is as a visual aid. If you are training other nurses, using a tablet to show images or related video can really help bring the point home. If you have a hospital-provided tablet and available images or video, a tablet can also be useful in explaining procedures to patients. It's one thing to hand out pamphlets or flyers about a topic, but using a tablet to show video or even interactive content is quite another. You can really increase your audience's interest if you make your presentation more entertaining and digitally focused.

MAC VS. PC

In the world of nerds, Macs and PCs are constantly compared. Each side has its strong supporters offering legitimate reasons why one is better than another. It's kind of like Democrats and Republicans. Apple products are on the rise, and it's reported that half of U.S. households own at least one Apple device (iPhone, iPad, Mac). Mac owners are typically male, have higher incomes, and are college educated. About a million jokes go along with whether you are a Mac or a PC user, but I won't bore you. The Internet is full of examples—just Google to your heart's content.

If you aren't already using a PC daily, you may find that a Mac is a bit more intuitive. It has subtle differences in functionality, such as a single mouse button, compared to two on a PC. This means there is no right-click option, so if you are accustomed to using the right button of the mouse while using a PC, then you may feel like something is missing when you use a Mac. This was one of my personal experiences and is often one of the biggest hurdles that Mac converts have to face.

There is also a different operating system, which many find to be easier to navigate. The built-in photo editing and video editing tools are great, and if you've ever wanted to create professional-looking home movies, then a Mac is where it's at.

Macs really shine in the creative areas. They include many intuitive and powerful graphic/design, music, and video editing tools. Some of the programs are quite expensive, but many professionals swear by Macs specifically for the speed and reliability they experience while using these apps. Many media apps come free with a Mac, such as iTunes, iPhoto, iMovie, and iDVD, and others are quite affordable.

If you ask Mac users why they prefer a Mac to a PC, they will probably tell you, "It just works." Macs are designed in such a way that they almost intuitively meet the needs of most consumers.

IS THE CHOICE EASY?

They say once you go Mac, you never go back, but I can tell you from personal experience that that is totally whack. Although I am a PC owner, I am a huge fan of Apple products. Personally, I own an Apple iPad and iPhone and believe that in terms of mobile operating systems, they are superior. With actual computer systems, it is really a matter of personal preference. I know many nurses and non-nurses alike who purchase Macs exclusively. They've owned them for years and have had better success with them than their PC counterparts. The only time that I feel myself wanting a Mac is when I'm at a conference or some other type of event, and I'm sitting in a room full of Macs. The design of a MacBook Pro is so beautiful and elegant that it's hard not to look down at your PC laptop, whose appearance is downright drab in comparison, and be jealous of the Mac's styling.

Macs also typically fare much better in the world of viruses. Although it's not impossible for Macs to become infected with viruses and spyware, it is far less common than in PCs. If you do not want to do a great deal of maintenance to your computer system, then a Mac may be a better choice for you.

Many programs have been created for Macs, and a large community of developers is making apps specially programmed in the operating system's language, which makes them very fast. Apple reviews apps that go into its marketplace, which keeps the quality higher than many PC apps. Many familiar programs, such as Microsoft Office, are available for Macs as well.

Apple meticulously screens its hardware components and only allows certain types of hardware to be included in its computers. This makes the initial purchase and upgrades more expensive but usually ensures that the system overall works much more reliably. Because the hardware is more propriety, make sure that any additional hardware (printers, extra memory, protable storage) that you buy for your Mac computer has been Apple approved.

Windows-based PCs are what you will find on most hospital networks, because most software vendors create their software to run on Windows computers and Windows servers. IT professionals agree that working in a Windows-based environment is much easier than attempting to repair Macs and far less costly. If you're looking for a solution to outfit a practice, hospital, or your home, PCs are going to offer you the best bang for your buck initially and be much easier on your wallet if you run into a problem with them.

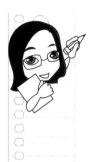

NERDY NOTE

A server is like a supercomputer that houses large amounts of data, program files, settings, and other information needed. This is where the patient records are ultimately stored.

The network is the connection that the computers have within the hospital. This can be an intranet (internal to the hospital only) or an extranet (allowing access to the Internet).

One of the biggest benefits that Windows has going for it is its strong developer base. More programmers know how to create programs in a Windows environment than in any other. This is why you see a greater variety of software available for PC, with better support and more competition.

Making the choice between a PC and a Mac is tough. I've tried both and believe that either of them can get the job done. Ultimately, you should go with your gut and buy the computer that speaks to you.

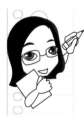

NERDY NOTE

It's also not a bad idea to buy the type of computer that your computer nerd friend likes. If you run into issues, a Mac advocate is much more likely to help you for free with a Mac issue.

COMPUTERS IN TVS, SERIOUSLY?

You may have seen advertisements for so-called smart TVs—heck, you may even own one. These TVs have integrated technology that allows you to access the Web through the TV to stream video, music, images, and even web pages. This feature usually adds several hundred dollars to the cost of a TV, but people really like the added benefits they get.

But what if you already have a perfectly good working TV and want to get in on all this smart TV action? Have no fear! Wireless streaming boxes are here!

Roku boxes and Apple TVs are amazing devices that can transform any HMDI-equipped TV into a high-tech marvel for less than $100. These devices are about the size of a small slice of bread and pack some pretty impressive computer components inside. They connect to your home's wireless network and allow you to access popular video-streaming services. Roku even gives you the ability to check out Facebook and play games like Angry Birds.

Apple TV is a smart TV solution produced by the same company that brought you the iPhone. It integrates popular streaming services like Netflix, Hulu Plus, and YouTube. You also get the ability to rent or purchase content directly from iTunes. Most experts argue that Apple TV is lacking in streaming content choices, but what it lacks in streaming capabilities, it makes up for with Airplay.

Airplay is amazing technology that allows you to stream whatever is on the screen of your iPhone, iPad, or Mac to your TV screen. It really takes gaming, streaming video, and sharing media with friends or family to a whole new level. After watching YouTube videos on the big screen, I can attest to the fact that Apple TV made something spectacular with Airplay technology.

TECH TIP

In order for Airplay to work, your devices need to be connected to the same wireless network. Sorry if this ruined any of your plans to take over the TV while you were away from home.

Roku is the second-most-popular streaming device, but it offers significantly more choices in streaming content, the ability to share and locate content via a USB device, and even the ability to play games (in some models). The channel lineup is growing daily and already offers more than 750 streaming channels. Netflix and Hulu are in the mix, of course, but you also get great streaming choices through Amazon Instant Video, HBO GO, PBS, Disney, Crackle, and Blockbuster, just to name a few.

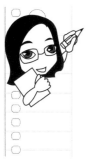

NERDY NOTE

Have you ever heard of Crackle? It's a really cool and free streaming service available via smartphone, tablet, and computer. It features some pretty good movies and TV shows, but unlike other services, like Netflix and Hulu, Crackle is completely free.

So what kind of movies does it offer? Well, I found *The Fifth Element* on there and then stopped looking. If it has one the best movies of all time for free, then I know it's good stuff!

TAKE ME OUT OF THE OVEN, I'M DONE!

OK, so we're not totally done, but we are wrapping up this chapter. We went over a lot, so I hope you paid attention. There's a quiz? What, you didn't study? It's a good thing this is open book then:

+ List a few keyboard shortcuts that can speed up your documentation time.

+ Which feature that Apple TV includes makes it really attractive for people who already own Apple products?

+ What should you do if the devices you are using to document patient care are not efficient or are difficult to use?

+ How can you disinfect a tablet?

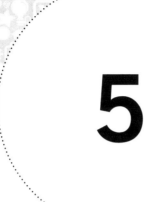

5

GETTING SMART ABOUT SMARTPHONES

Sam Morse and Alexander Graham Bell would be amazed at how far we have come in communication technology. We are no longer burdened with wires and landlines. Many consumers have chosen to abandon traditional home phones altogether and instead opt to use only cell phones. It is difficult to comprehend that in the not-too-distant past, we marveled at our ability to carry a cellular phone and make calls while away from home. However, technology has rapidly advanced, and what started as bulky units with monochrome screens and minimal functions have progressed to full-fledged pocket computers with sophisticated graphic interfaces.

I've known several nurses who never thought they'd want a smartphone, but for one reason or another, they ended up purchasing one. Now most of them can't begin to comprehend what they did before they had smartphones. This is especially obvious when they try to go back to texting on a regular cell phone.

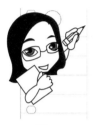

NERDY NOTE

If you want a quick response from someone, text message is sometimes the best method. If you are trying to get ahold of someone who is in a meeting or unable to talk on the phone, the person may be able to answer a text.

I know some nurses who work in home care who finally received agency-provided cell phones, but there was a catch! They were just regular old cell phones. The nurses were happy to have these phones, but the number one complaint from every nurse was "It's really hard to text on one." Most of the nurses had upgraded to smartphones on their personal lines and were really missing their keyboard features.

CODE CAUTION

Standard text messages are not secure! Do not under any circumstances send PHI through a text message.

Technology usually follows the "You don't know what you are missing" rule. Even if you know something exists, until you experience it, you really don't miss it. The luxury of a nice smartphone may not be needed, but it can certainly make your life easier. And it can even be a great job aid for nurses.

In this chapter, I discuss how nurses can use smartphones on the job. I also talk a little bit about the different types of smartphones, operating systems, carriers, and hardware. If you're really awesome and ask really nicely, I might even suggest some helpful apps for your smartphone!

Because technology is good for work and play, let's touch on a little of both.

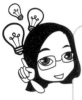

TECH TIP

You might often hear the terms "hardware" and "software" when it comes to technology, but you might be a little confused about the difference.

Hardware refers to the actual device itself. This might be a computer, smartphone, or digital camera.

Software refers to the programming language that allows a piece of hardware to operate. This can be anything from Windows to Adobe.

Hardware and software must work together for you to have functioning technology.

SMARTPHONES FOR NURSING?

Nurses can use smartphones in a variety of ways. You can use apps to help you get more information about medications or diseases. You can look up videos about procedures on YouTube. You can also use apps to gain CE credits, which is a licensure requirement of many states.

For many, having a smartphone gives them a sense of security and safety by allowing them to stay connected. You can also use your smartphone to keep you informed. The handy calendar apps and other productivity tools available on a smartphone can really help you to stay organized and on track.

TECH TIP

Some really great document storage apps like JotNot! Scan are excellent for storing copies of your important documents in your smartphone. You can have your BLS card and your nursing license in your pocket at all times!

STAYING CONNECTED

It wasn't too long ago that having a mobile phone of any kind was a luxury that most couldn't afford. Technology has improved at a blazing rate and has accordingly decreased the cost of owning mobile technology to the level where most consumers can afford it. Smartphones build on this technology and give you even more ways to stay connected.

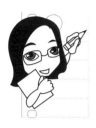

NERDY NOTE

Smartphones have become very affordable. You can pick up some really nice Windows phones for *free* with a 2-year contract.

Many may worry that having smartphones might be a potential distraction for nurses. This concern is valid, and nurses need to be aware of the potential for abuse and misuse. To avoid any instances of improper use in the workplace, employers of nurses should be clear on their smartphone policies. However, a simple "no mobile phones in patient care areas" edict is really going a bit too far. If you eliminate the use of smartphones during patient care, you are eliminating the many benefits they can offer to nurses. If your employer has taken this hard stand against smartphones, I strongly encourage you to present management with examples of the many benefits of using a smartphone while on the floor.

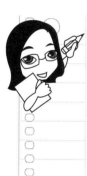

NERDY NOTE

If your employer has a "no smartphone" policy, I am not suggesting that you break the rules. What I do suggest is that you question the policy and by doing so advocate for yourself and your patients. Many articles support using smartphones and evidence-based practice nursing through medical apps during patient care (Mosa, Yoo, & Sheets, 2012). Show these articles, and possibly this book, to management to win them over.

Nurses are on the front lines of health care and are usually in areas with large populations of people. A hospital could be a prime target for a terrorist attack, and it's important that nurses be able to communicate with their families. This extra sense of security can make doing a difficult job a little less stressful.

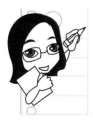

NERDY NOTE

Some hospitals use hospital-owned smartphones as their means of communicating with their nurses. Instead of carrying a regular cordless phone or a pager, each nurse instead carries a smartphone. The nerd in me thinks this development is awesome!

STAYING INFORMED

Nurses can use smartphones to stay informed on a variety of topics ranging from nursing-related issues to the local weather. This information can be helpful for nurses in many ways.

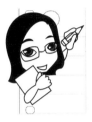

NERDY NOTE

Don't think the weather is important? Check your hospital's attendance policy—most require that you report to work even during a snowstorm. It's useful to know about these things ahead of time, and smartphones can give you a heads-up.

Nurses need to stay up to date on current events related to changes in health care and even broad-reaching health events that might be taking place. If smartphones were around a hundred years ago, the influenza epidemic of 1918 could have possibly been avoided. Imagine if there were pandemic flu quarantine apps that notified you if a patient had been infected in your area. Think of the potential lifesaving ability that a single app could have in the right hands.

Because many experts claim that we are due for another epidemic, it would be useful for all nurses to have smartphones. Imagine if the Centers for Disease Control and Prevention (CDC) sent alerts to you, and you could instantly know whether the next major outbreak had reached your area. You could know when to wear a mask or other protective gear and potentially save thousands of lives.

The future is actually closer than you might think—the CDC has already created a pretty amazing smartphone app called FluView that tracks flulike illness and alerts you of the activity. Check out the CDC's website for more information and download the app on a smartphone near you.

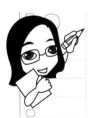

NERDY NOTE

Several apps tracked the progression of the swine flu.

You can also use a smartphone to stay informed about health care laws and regulations. Although many nurses believe that this responsibility is above their pay grade, it is helpful for all nurses to be aware of the standards their employers are held to. After all, nurses will be doing most of the work by performing patient care on the front lines, and practicing within the scope of your license is your responsibility and no one else's.

Another thing to consider is that many nurses are also involved in creating these laws and regulations. Any number of you who are reading this book right now could be policymakers and have the ability to affect nurses and patients on a grand scale. If you're going to be making and enforcing rules, it is extremely important to stay current on technology and have quick and convenient access to information.

STAYING ON SCHEDULE

Many useful apps and tools are available for smartphones to help you stay on schedule. One of the most basic apps is a calendar. With many nurses taking extra shifts and getting paid overtime, it's important for them to keep track of all the time they've worked. If you are in this situation, you need to make sure you know when you have to be at work, but you also need to make sure you are being paid for all the time you have put in.

You can also use your smartphone to create task lists and help you improve your time-management skills. You can write quick notes to yourself or record brief voice memos to quickly remember things.

CODE CAUTION

You should be aware that if you are using your personal smartphone, you should not include any identifiable patient information on your personal device. There are many reasons for this, first and foremost being that your personal device is not encrypted.

PURCHASING A SMARTPHONE

If you don't already own a smartphone but you've decided to purchase one, you'll want to make sure you're getting a mobile device that will meet all your needs. Going to the cell phone store and just picking one out may leave you feeling disappointed. To be completely honest, you're likely to be directed to a phone based upon the preferences of the salesperson rather than your own. Spend some time researching your options prior to purchasing a smartphone to determine which one is right for you.

Let me be upfront with you and say that my preferred smartphone is an iPhone. I've had one for years and can't imagine my life without it. I've used others types of smartphones and am often unimpressed or confused by how they work (and I'm a nerd). Because I consider myself to be very technologically inclined, if a phone intimidates me, then it will likely intimidate others. The iPhone has never disappointed me and always "just works." If you sense this bias in the following pages, now you'll understand why.

This doesn't mean, however, that an iPhone is right for everyone. It's up to you to decide which device meets your needs. You should weigh the pros and cons of all the models available and pick the one that fits your budget and your lifestyle. Test it out thoroughly within the first few days of ownership, and if it doesn't meet your needs, take advantage of the 14-day return policy that most carriers offer.

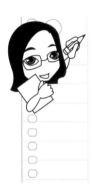

NERDY NOTE

Most people stick with the type of smartphone they buy. If you start with an Android, you are probably always going to use an Android. You'll upgrade, of course, but once you get used to the environment, it's just inconvenient to switch. You should also know that once you've purchased apps, music, or any other content, it is not transferrable to a different apps store. For example, if you buy songs from the Android marketplace, you would have to buy them *again* through the iTunes stores if you wanted to switch to an iPhone.

OPERATING SYSTEM LOWDOWN

Because smartphones are tiny computers, it should come as little surprise that they come with many different operating systems (OS). OS refers to the core software of the device that is responsible for the feel and interface of the phone and provides the backbone for its functions. Although most smartphones operate similarly, their OSs can create subtle differences. Many users do notice these differences and often develop a preference.

In the nerd community, lively debates rage on regarding which is the *better* smartphone, but what I've come to realize is that they really are all about the same. The differences between gestures and app marketplaces are noticeable, but only when you have a basis for comparison. Generally speaking, whichever smartphone OS you start with is probably the one you will like the best. You will get used to your phone operating a certain way and anything different will seem subpar, even if it does exactly the same thing.

But to give you a little better insight into the world of smartphones, let's take a brief look at the most popular operating systems, brands, wireless carriers, and even a few apps. Ultimately, your decision of which smartphone to buy is probably going to be greatly influenced by the phones that your friends and family have. It's a good idea to find a friend or coworker who can help you pick out a phone that is right for you and answer your questions along the way.

WHICH OS IS BEST?

The three main players in the smartphone market are Android, iOS, and Windows. Oh, there's also Blackberry, but I'm not even sure who is buying those anymore. Regardless, I could devote chapters and possibly even an entire book to the differences, but it's likely you already have one of these phones, and that's probably the one you're going to stick with. Once you get comfortable with a particular operating system, switching to a different one can be a burden.

When it comes to nursing, however, iPhone really tends to shine. Significantly more apps are available in Apple's App Store to help you do your job. This is followed by Android, which offers a competitive amount of nursing apps. Windows drags in at third place. Blackberry— well, again, I don't even know who has one anymore. If you've got a Blackberry, I can't help you.

If you're picking up a new smartphone and aren't superimpressed with the one you currently have, my vote always goes to iPhone. Unless you've invested a ton of money in content like apps and music on your smartphone, it's worthwhile to make the switch.

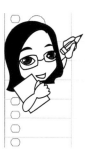

NERDY NOTE

It might sound like Apple is stuffing cash in my back pocket to give the company this glowing endorsement. Actually, Apple doesn't do that—it doesn't have to. The fans of Apple products sing their praises free of charge. Interestingly enough, Apple is one of the only major companies that doesn't employ lobbyists or even provide free products for tech analysts to review (trust me, I've tried).

WHAT ABOUT DEVICES?

Apple only produces the iPhone. A new version is released about once a year. Typically, Apple releases a model with major upgrades every 2 years. The major upgrade is usually designated with a number, like iPhone 4 or iPhone 5. The phone released a year after that typically has fewer impressive enhancements and has historically been named by adding an "S" to the model (i.e., iPhone 4S and iPhone 5S). These are the only phones that run on the iOS operating system.

NERDY NOTE

One of the most annoying things about being an iPhone user is how they are released. If you don't pick up the newest model within 3 months of its release, then you are better off waiting for the next release. Nothing is more frustrating than getting a brand-new iPhone only to have the newest model come out a month after you've picked yours up and sell for the same price! Pay attention to release dates, and always ask your salesperson when the next iPhone release is anticipated.

Generally speaking, an iPhone is released once a year. Sometimes this is 9 months after the last one, and sometimes it's more than 12.

If you've really got your heart set on getting an iPhone and want to know whether you should buy now or wait, you can check out some popular blogs that are devoted almost entirely to Apple and Mac rumors. MacRumors (www.macrumors.com), 9to5Mac (www.9to5mac.com), and The Unofficial Apple Weblog (www.tuaw.com) are just a few of the many locations on the Web where Mac nerds swoon over Apple innovations and share any leaks related to new Apple products. You might have to wade through some non-iPhone content, but if a new iPhone model is on the way, chances are pretty good that it will be discussed in at least one of these places.

Android phones are made by a variety of manufacturers. Samsung, HTC, Motorola, and LG are the most popular and make the highest-quality smartphones. The Samsung Galaxy and the Samsung Note are extremely popular models and usually among the best-selling. These are at the higher end of the price range of smartphones but offer attractive features like larger screens, higher screen resolution, and the most up-to-date version of Android.

Windows phones are made by Samsung, Nokia, and HTC. Fewer choices are available than with Android phones, but they still outnumber iPhone options. Oftentimes you can get a Windows phone with excellent features for a very low cost and possibly even free with a 2-year contract.

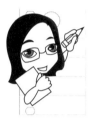

NERDY NOTE

I actually really like Windows phones. If I weren't already so heavily invested in iPhone apps and media, it would be on my radar.

Most cell phone service providers subsidize the price of your phone if you sign a 2-year contract. You may be apprehensive to sign a contract for a new phone, but you should consider the fact that you know that you are going to keep a phone, so you might as well save money on a new phone. Even if you bring your own phone to a provider, most of them require you to sign a contract for adding a new line of service.

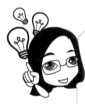

TECH TIP

Many organizations that employ nurses sign up with cell phone providers to give discounts to nurses. Check with your employer and your cell phone provider to see whether you are eligible for any discounts. My discount through my employer is 20% off the base plan, which really adds up over time.

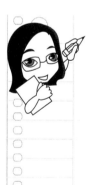

NERDY NOTE

Don't be apprehensive about signing a cell phone contract. You can always change the options in your plan by calling your cell phone provider or visiting a corporate location. I would recommend the phone route, because the retail stores can be pretty busy with long waits for service-related requests.

Most carriers also allow you to make adjustments to your phone plan on their websites. It's usually very easy to do, but if you have trouble, customer service is only a chat box or phone call away.

If you decide you want to switch carriers—say, from Verizon to AT&T—this can be accomplished as well. All you have to do is initiate new service with the provider of your choice in the store or over the phone. I personally recommend going to a corporate store (not an authorized reseller). Staff there will take care of most details for you, including terminating service on the other account, transferring your existing number to your new phone, and usually even importing your contacts into your new phone. You should be aware, however, that if you have time remaining in the original contract you signed, you will almost certainly be responsible for paying a hefty termination fee to your former carrier.

TECH TIP

If you tell a carrier that you have contract time remaining with another provider, the new carrier will often help offset the termination fee with a billing credit. I've had my first month's bill reduced by as much as $100 when I switched carriers.

WHICH WIRELESS CARRIER ROCKS?

Once you have decided which smartphone you want to purchase, you also need to decide which cell phone carrier you want to be with. If you already have a feature phone (non-smartphone cell phone), then you may already be satisfied with your service, but take some time to research the coverage in your area and determine which type of data plan you are going to get.

Many providers offer phones on a contract basis: If you agree to use their service for a period of years, they will offer you a new smartphone at a significantly discounted rate. Through these discounts, most popular smartphones are less than $200, and some of them are even free!

CNET is a popular technology-review and consumer-focused website that offers a guide to comparing phone carriers (German, 2013). CNET recommends that you compare the following features in carriers:

1. Coverage

2. Data speeds

3. Plans

4. Your phone

5. Customer service

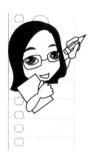

NERDY NOTE

Customer service experience can vary drastically from caller to caller. In the past, I've felt that Verizon had superior customer service, but now I believe that the overall service from AT&T is better. Ultimately, if you aren't getting the level of service that you think is appropriate, you should ask for a supervisor. This usually makes the call go much more smoothly.

COMPARING MAJOR WIRELESS NETWORKS

It can be difficult to stay up to date on the offerings of the wireless carriers. They frequently change the programs and promotions they offer, but the pricing is usually fairly comparable and varies by about $20 a month, depending on the carrier. What you will notice is that not all the providers offer unlimited data. This is a selling point for many high-demand smart-phone users but is really not a major concern for most.

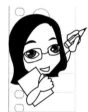

NERDY NOTE

Remember to factor in that discount you get from your employer. Being a nurse can actually save you money in this instance!

Although most users prefer to have an unlimited data plan, Verizon and AT&T no longer offer this feature. If you've been grandfathered in on an old AT&T plan, you can keep your unlimited data, but Verizon forces you to choose a shared (and limited) data plan if you want to upgrade your phone. This has been a sore subject among many smartphone users, but unfortunately AT&T and Verizon have shown no signs of bringing unlimited data back.

My nerd rage sometimes gets the best of me on this topic, because I cling to my unlimited data plan and really feel chained to my provider (AT&T) because of it. Honestly, though, I've had excellent customer service from AT&T, so I can't complain. There is the small grievance of throttling, or limiting your speed, after using a certain portion of data. Because I usually don't reach the threshold, this isn't a big deal.

NERDY NOTE

Although I do have an unlimited data plan and would feel practically naked without it, I rarely use more than 2GB of data a month. My Nerdy Nurse advice is not to stress over the amount of data in your plan. Chances are you will never get close to your limit.

However, it is worth mentioning that if you have a shared data plan, you should probably pay closer attention to your data usage. Although you may not use a ton of data, you might have a teenager or husband who is heavily into music and media streaming. This activity can eat up all your bandwidth and leave you vulnerable to hefty overage fees or throttling. Make sure all users are aware of when they are and aren't on a Wi-Fi connection and to monitor their data use accordingly.

Pricing and unlimited data aside, you should really compare the coverage area where you live. Each wireless carrier offers a coverage map, although I recommend that you take these with a grain of salt. Even though an area may show up as "good" coverage, if your house is in a valley, has a mountain nearby, or lies near any other large obstruction, chances are that you could be in a "dead spot." A good idea is to ask your neighbors who their wireless service providers are and whether they are satisfied with their cell phone reception. Also, most carriers allow you to return a phone and cancel any contract if you test out the device/coverage and are not satisfied within the first 14 days.

If you work out in the field as a home care nurse, then having reliable cell phone service is really important. Although most users agree that Verizon has the best coverage in rural areas, some places in the hills of Georgia and Alabama prevent even the best service provider from guaranteeing coverage.

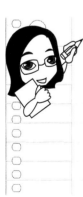

NERDY NOTE

If you live in an area that doesn't have good coverage but you really like your carrier otherwise, you can always get a microcell. These are small devices that are about the size of a router that transform your broadband Internet service into a cell phone signal and pretty much eliminate any dropped calls at home. These can be picked up online or at your local wireless carrier retail store. If you no longer have a home phone and are required to be on call for your job, a wireless microcell is a great way to ensure you get every call.

Table 4.1   Wireless carrier comparison

VERIZON	AT&T	SPRINT	T-MOBILE
4G LTE	4G LTE	4G LTE	4G LTE
CDMA	GSM	CDMA	GSM
"Share Everything" Plan: unlimited text/ calls, sharing a limited amount of data	Shared data plans or individual data plans per phone	Flat rate unlimited data/text, and 1,500-minute calling plans	Value plans can include unlimited data, text, and calling
Family plans	Family plans	Family plans	Family plans
Prepaid available	Prepaid available	Prepaid available	Prepaid available

TECH TIP

CDMA and GSM are the types of wireless signals that cell phone carriers use. A lot of technical jargon would go into explaining the differences, but three key things stand out: (1) GSM is the most widely used format, and if you travel the world, your phone is more likely to work abroad if you have a GSM phone; (2) GSM phones support the ability to surf the Web and talk at the same time, and although you may be asking who wants to do that, I can promise you that there will come a time when you want to look something up while talking on the phone; and (3) CDMA is said to be more secure and to reduce the number of dropped calls experienced by users.

If you are unsure which carrier to go with, Table 4.1 should give you the information you need to compare CDMA and GSM.

TRAVELING WITH A SMARTPHONE

Something that should be taken into consideration when deciding which network you wish to purchase your smartphone on is how often you plan to travel. Depending on where you plan to go, your smartphone may or may not work. For example, Sprint coverage is usually great in major cities but decreases as you enter more rural areas.

If you plan to travel to Europe or South America several times, then you might want to consider a smartphone that uses GSM technology (AT&T or T-Mobile). You can switch out your SIM card while you are abroad and still use your device. If you are not planning on frequenting other countries (or just don't want to be contacted once you get there), then using a GSM wireless carrier isn't really as important.

TECH TIP

A SIM card (subscriber identity module) gives life to your mobile device. It identifies the phone as belonging to you and allows it to authenticate and connect to a wireless network. If wireless carriers are the gatekeepers, then SIM cards are the keymasters.

Having a cell phone that can potentially work anywhere can be a major benefit to nurses. If you've ever considered working in disaster relief, then it's important that you have a cell phone that can function wherever you go. Or perhaps you or your spouse is a member of the military and is constantly traveling nationally and abroad. It would be very inconvenient to switch out your entire phone every few months but very easy to just pop in a new SIM card when you got to a new location. This way all your nursing apps, contacts, appointments, and customization would remain the same, but you would still be able to stay connected.

TECH TIP

If you're going to be away from work for any period of time, you might want to consider setting up your work email on your device. This is usually accomplished by going into the settings of your phone and adding a new mail account. Although setting up email on your smartphone is usually pretty straightforward, when it comes to work email accounts, there is a little more involved. Each employer has different settings related to its network, so it's best if you contact your IT department for guidance. If your employer allows you to check work email remotely, someone in IT will be happy to walk you through the setup process.

WHAT'S UP WITH APPS?

Apps are one of the biggest draws of smartphone ownership. Each operating system has its own app store, and apps offer software to do many simple and complex tasks. There are apps for social media networks, word processing, sharing documents and media, managing finances, photo editing, and so much more. You could spend hours just browsing your phone's app store and finding new and interesting apps.

TECH TIP

Did you know that many new apps are created every day? In a few spare moments, you can check out the "Hot" or "New" section of your app marketplace to find some cool, neat apps that will put you on the cutting edge of mobile technology.

You could also spend hours finding utterly useless and completely overpriced apps. For instance, a large number of apps are devoted to bodily functions and the various noises they make—seriously. There are also apps that are meant purely to signify your status and come with equally ridiculous price tags. Although it's now been removed from Apple's App Store, the "I Am Rich" app boasted a $999 price tag and did nothing at all. If you're interested in keeping up with the frequency of your bowel movements, there is even an app for you! For a mere $0.99, "Poo Log" gives you a timer and a journal with which to keep track of this lovely little detail of your life. Although I'm sure GI nurses everywhere will probably find this highly amusing, I am sure this information could be gathered without the $0.99 price tag.

Knowing that there are some truly ridiculous apps available is helpful so you know to avoid them. If you're curious about whether an app is worth investing in, either monetarily or in digital real estate, Google reviews of the app to find out what you need to know.

Many useful apps are completely free and don't even include any form of advertising. Other apps may run small advertisements or be available for a small price (typically $0.99). At the time of this publication, Apple's App Store has more apps available than any other app marketplace, with more than 900,000. The Google Play Store for Android devices boasts more than 650,000, while the Windows phone store lags yet still has more than 150,000 apps available.

Most of the apps that are referenced on the following pages are available in multiple app stores.

FINANCIAL

✢ **Mint:** (FREE) It is easier than ever to track your financial status. Mint allows you to link all your financial accounts so that you can see your current financial situation. It even helps you keep up with balances on your checking accounts and updates automatically.

✢ **Manilla:** (FREE) This app helps you keep track of when your bills are due and allows you to pay them directly within the app.

✢ **Online Banking:** (FREE) Many larger banks like Synovus and Chase offer specific apps that let you track your purchases and transfer funds, and some even allow you to deposit checks electronically just by taking a picture with your smartphone.

NURSING

✢ **iTriage:** (FREE) This app features many excellent tools for nurses and patients alike. Patients can use it to help determine whether they need to seek medical care. Nurses can use it to explain medical procedures, review medications, and provide education to patients.

✢ **Epocrates Essentials:** (FREE) This is a very useful app for nurses at all levels of experience. Its drug reference library includes entries for herbals and over-the-counter (OTC) medications as well as a pill identifier. It also has useful information on disease and lab test references.

✢ **Medscape:** (FREE) If you are looking for the latest medical news, then this app has you covered. It also lets you research medications, procedures, and medical conditions. I've found this app really helpful when researching the latest news regarding diseases and standards.

✢ **Davis's Drug Guide:** ($39.99) This is one of the most popular drug guides for nurses and is even better in mobile format. It is a little more expensive than other apps, but many nurses agree that it's worth the price.

✢ **Pocket Lab Values:** ($2.99) This is a great app for helping you keep track of lab values. It also allows you to edit certain details like tube colors to match the policies of your facility. It gives details about the values, differential diagnoses, details on why labs may be ordered, and so much more.

✛ **Nursing Central:** (FREE) This app includes many useful reference materials for nurses, including information related to diseases, nursing diagnoses, and medical diagnoses.

✛ **Resuscitation!:** (FREE) This innovative simulation app puts you in charge of a patient's care during a critical situation. Although in the game you play "doctor," it's a great way to hone your knowledge and reaction to emergency situations.

MUSIC

✛ **Pandora:** (FREE) This app gives you the ability to listen to music for free. It has limited interruptions and allows you to indicate whether you like or dislike songs to build music channels specific to your interests.

TECH TIP

Most of these apps have free and premium versions. If you're really into music, it might be worth investing a few dollars a month to have more control over the music you hear.

✛ **Spotify:** (FREE) This is a subscription-based music app that allows you to listen to almost any song or album you can think of. You are essentially renting the music and can listen to whatever you want as often as you want for as long as you are paying the low monthly fee. Some of the features can be accessed for free, but if you want instant on-demand access to any song, then you will have to pay the subscription fee. If you'd like to test it first to decide whether it's worth it, the desktop version allows more functionality for *free*!

✛ **iHeartRadio:** (FREE) This app allows you to listen to various radio stations across the United States. You can also create your own custom music channels based upon your interests.

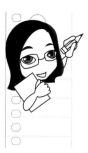

NERDY NOTE

Music plays a big role in the life of many nurses. Whether you are pumping up the volume to get amped for a shift or playing some relaxing music to unwind, you've got to have music! Some nurses, like those who work in home health care or behind the scenes in administration, may even have the opportunity to listen to music while they work. This can really make the day go by faster and reduce your stress level.

NAVIGATION

+ **NAVIGON:** ($39.99) This pay app features accurate directions and text-to-speech technology. It has integrated Google maps images and shows you what your destination should look like on screen. This app is a bit costly, but it's one of the best navigation apps I've ever used. If you want excellent traffic updates while you're trying to get across town to check on your home care patient, this is a great app to use.

+ **Waze:** (FREE) This is a unique crowd-sourced navigation app that relies on data from its users to improve its maps. It also reports traffic situations and accidents based upon the speed cars are traveling and direct user reports.

+ **MapQuest:** (FREE) This app is easy to use and is generally reliable. It allows customization and gives turn-by-turn audio and visual directions.

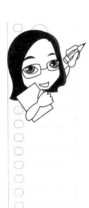

NERDY NOTE

Crowdsourcing is a fairly new concept online, but it basically allows technologies to be improved by getting input from many. Every time you use the Waze app, you are actually helping improve its maps. It also automatically reports slowdowns instantly, so that others using Waze are warned when there is heavy traffic or an accident in the area. This type of information helps ensure that you get to your shift on time, and it's kind of cool to think that you can help others by just driving and using this app. It's like getting to take care of patients without even having to do anything out of the ordinary.

VIDEOS AND MOVIES

+ **Netflix:** (FREE) This subscription-based service works on computers and TVs and has a smartphone app. You can watch as many movies and television shows as you want for a small monthly fee.

+ **YouTube:** (FREE) This app allows you to watch YouTube videos on the go. Whether you need a laugh or want to learn more about a particular topic, YouTube is a welcome addition to any smartphone.

+ **Individual TV providers:** (FREE) Many television providers, including Comcast and AT&T U-verse, offer their own smartphone apps. These apps often let you access your DVR and play on demand content on your mobile device. It usually also acts as a remote control.

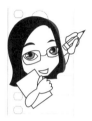

NERDY NOTE

You could watch many great health care documentaries and nursing films via these services—or you could also just watch some really bad reality TV and destress after a tough shift. You eat, sleep, and breathe patient care for a large portion of your life, so sometimes it's just nice to sit back and relax.

UTILITIES

+ **RoboForm:** (FREE–$19.99) This is an excellent app that helps you manage your passwords. It can be used in conjunction with PC- or Mac-based applications and gives you access to your passwords while on the go.

+ **JotNot! Pro:** ($1.99) This is a useful app for helping you track important documents and receipts. You can use your smartphone's camera to capture images of these documents, file them, or send them to your cloud storage accounts or email addresses. This is a great way to keep your nursing license, certifications, and CEs handy. If anyone ever needs a copy of them, you can just email them right from the app!

+ **OneNote:** (FREE) This app allows you to organize notes and separate them into notebooks. It also has the ability to sync with an online Microsoft account.

+ **Evernote:** (FREE) This is a great app that can help you organize your life. Whether you are planning a health fair, cataloging your favorite recipes, or doing best practice research, this app, in conjunction with the desktop version, keeps everything sorted.

These are by no means inclusive lists, but they are leaping off points to get you started on your very own app journey. There are apps for cooking, gaming, news, social media, travel planning, home remodeling, learning, humor, and so much more. It's hard to even think about how many devices your smartphone has replaced. It's an amazing piece of technology that has really revolutionized how we live, communicate, and if you let it, provide patient care.

ARE YOU SMART ABOUT SMARTPHONES YET?

This has been quite a chapter hasn't it? By now you should feel just about as smart as that smartphone in your pocket—or at least competent enough to browse through the app stores for a few new apps.

Did you pay attention? Here's a quiz:

✦ What is the difference between GSM and CDMA?

✦ How do you set up your work email on your smartphone?

✦ Which app helps you with lab values?

Five chapters down and four more to go. You can do this!

REFERENCES

German, K. (2013, February 7). Quick guide to cell phone carriers. *CNET*. Retrieved from http://reviews.cnet.com/best-cell-phone-carriers/

Mosa, A. S. M., Yoo, I., & Sheets, L. (2012, July). A systematic review of healthcare applications for smartphones. *BMC Medical Informatics and Decision Making, 12*, 67. Retrieved from http://link.springer.com/article/10.1186/1472-6947-12-67#

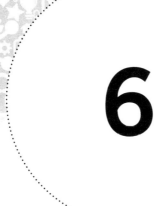

6

TABLETS ARE YOUR NEW BEST FRIEND

Health care is constantly changing and evolving. With every new innovation in technology, nursing and patient care stand to benefit. Tablets are an excellent example of an innovation that changes the way we interact with technology on a daily basis. Tablets are humanizing technology and making digital content more accessible and often more favorable than traditional print media. The benefits we could gain from the use of tablets are only just now becoming evident.

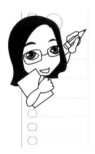

NERDY NOTE

Humanizing technology is important. It helps to make it more familiar and easier to adapt to. For most, it's much easier to talk to a person than it is to understand the complex workings of a computer. Tablets simplify things and destress the process of using technology. Unless you're a hardcore nerd like me, this simplification is welcome.

Tablets are similar to smartphones and often use many of the same apps. Depending on the tablet you are using, it may include a camera, wireless broadband connectivity, and perhaps even wireless accessories, such as keyboards and other input devices. Each model has features that can be beneficial for work as well as for pleasure and can be used in some way to increase your skills as a nurse and improve the patient care you deliver.

TECH TIP

Although tablets usually don't come with wireless keyboards and other accessories in the box, most have the ability to pair with Bluetooth keyboards. These generally cost between $30 and $100 and can really help improve your productivity, especially if you are going to be using a tablet in the work setting to document lengthy patient notes.

Many health care organizations use tablets as a primary means for the nurses to interact with the patients' electronic medical records (EMRs). If done correctly, this can be a really great and intuitive experience for both the nurse and the patient. Tablets are usually even more portable than laptops and considerably more lightweight. This added freedom means that a nurse isn't constantly searching for a table to set the device down on and can use it more like a clipboard.

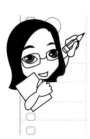

NERDY NOTE

Some really forward-thinking health care facilities even provide tablets to check patients in and have them complete any necessary insurance forms. This really can help eliminate a lot of duplicate work, and most patients think this sort of thing is cool and innovative.

In this chapter, I dive deeply into tablets. I discuss some basics about the different types of tablets and which features work well for nurses. I also talk about accessories that can help protect your tablet and make ownership much more enjoyable. And then I wrap things up with examples of how tablets can improve health care and nursing.

If you're reading this book on a tablet, then you've already got a head start here!

EASING YOURSELF INTO TECHNOLOGY

An easy way to slowly submerge yourself into the seemingly overwhelming sea of technology is to purchase a tablet. With a tablet, you'll find that many of the distracting and daunting tasks related to owning a traditional computer are virtually eliminated. Tablets are primarily devices designed for consuming content rather than producing it, and consequently they offer a much higher satisfaction rate.

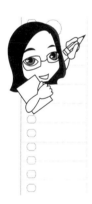

NERDY NOTE

Having a tablet at home is especially helpful if you are expected to use one at work. Although you should never feel pressured to buy the same device that you use at work, if you want to be really comfortable using it, then it couldn't hurt.

Although, if you use some insanely expensive Toughbook or medical-only device at work, you should refrain from purchasing a similar device for home use. However, it might be helpful to use something at home that runs on the same operating system.

We are all consumers. We consume goods and services. But often technology forces us to be creators as well. As fantastic and beneficial as the ability to create is, sometimes it also necessitates interaction that many of us would like to avoid. Computers are often overwhelming to many because they require input to be beneficial. Tablets, on the other hand, require very little input to yield results.

For nurses, tablets work well when the apps and interface they use keep patients in mind. If you are expected to complete lengthy text boxes, then a tablet is less than ideal. However, a series of questions with radio buttons or drop-down menus can be easily completed in a few taps on a tablet computer. Your patients will appreciate the fact that the technology is not getting in the way of the care you are giving, and you won't constantly be searching for a desk.

YOU'RE A CONSUMER, YOU NEED A CONSUMPTION DEVICE

Again, we are consumers. And tablets are consumption devices. They allow us to view content almost effortlessly—some might even say magically. Rather than requiring a keyboard, mouse, and navigation of a complex operating system (OS), tablets require little more than a few finger swipes to bring the information of the world into the palm of our hands.

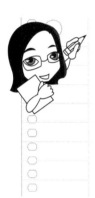

NERDY NOTE

If you are a patient educator, then tablets can be a really awesome tool for you. You can pull patient information up and sit at the person's bedside to share this information with the patient. On the very same device, you can show images, video, and other forms of education materials.

If the patient has an email address and your hospital policy allows it, you could email the educational information to the person rather than providing paper handouts that can easily be lost.

Which type of content is available for consumption on a tablet? A few examples of what you can view on a tablet include:

+ Images

+ Books

+ Music

+ Movies

+ Web pages

+ Emails

+ Games

+ Other forms of media

This content is available in a variety of forms ranging from web pages to files to apps. The amount of health care and nursing content available is growing every day, as are the means to access it. Tablets actually can help make this content more accessible because of their compact and portable nature. It's much easier to take a tablet out to quickly read a nursing article than it is to boot up the laptop.

HOW IS USING A TABLET DIFFERENT FROM USING A COMPUTER?

Using a traditional computer can be quite demanding. They can require a lot of work and know-how to get things done on them. Even if you only use a computer at work to chart on your patients, you know how frustrating they can be due to the numbers of clicks and steps required to complete simple tasks. Even something as simple as checking email is a process that takes time to understand specifically.

Tablets, on the other hand, require far less effort to get the same results because of the way you interact with them. Rather than dragging a mouse across the screen to click on an icon, you simply touch an icon. By changing the way you interact with this technology, the engineers behind tablet technology have already eliminated extraneous pieces and steps in the process. In nursing, we all have tricks to make processes simple and more streamlined. These time-savers work well because they simplify tasks we perform routinely. Tablets work the same way—they simplify the way we interact with digital content, providing a much more enjoyable and less daunting experience than traditional forms of computing offer.

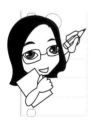

NERDY NOTE
Nursing already has enough complexity. Anything that can help simplify things is welcomed by most nurses.

WHAT'S THE DIFFERENCE BETWEEN TABLETS?

Here are a few questions you may be asking yourself already about owning a tablet:

✛ Why does the iPad retail for $499 while the Kindle Fire's price point is a much lower $199?

✦ What about the $49 tablet my friend bought off eBay?

✦ What's an Android tablet? Do I want one of those?

I'm happy to answer these questions and discuss the differences among several of the tablets available on the market today. As a nurse, you can use your tablet for both your personal and professional endeavors, and this chapter touches on how you can navigate the world of tablets so that you can feel confident about purchasing and owning one. Your ability to access information more easily as well as your improved comfort level with technology will help improve the quality of patient care you deliver. If you factor in the added ability to expand your nursing knowledge and add to your patient education, then you can clearly see the benefits of tablet ownership as a nurse.

FEATURES, APPS, AND OPERATING SYSTEMS

As with a computer or a car, you must consider many different models and features when you are looking at tablets. Features that you will want to investigate include screen size, screen input, design, battery life, storage and expansion, OS, apps selection, and available accessories.

SCREEN SIZE

Screen size and tablet size can be used almost interchangeably, because a tablet's size is defined primarily by its screen size. Tablets come in all shapes and sizes to fit a variety of different needs. Nurses might want tablets that are small and ultraportable to fit in their purses while they are on the go for personal use. But when they are at work, they might want larger screen real estate to display more patient data at once.

TECH TIP

When we talk about screen size, we are discussing the size measured from corner to corner diagonally. This is the industry standard measurement for screens and is also the way that flatscreen televisions are measured. This is a useful piece of technology information to know when shopping for many consumer electronics, such as tablets, TVs, and so forth.

RESISTIVE AND CAPACITIVE SCREENS

The type of screen that a tablet has determines the way you interact with it. It can also define your overall experience when consuming content. Capacitive screens respond to human touch because of the natural energy our body emits. Resistive screens respond to touch and pressure and are typically designed to receive their input from some form of stylus to give you the most enjoyable experience.

RESISTIVE SCREENS

Resistive touch screens respond to input based upon pressure and are often designed to work best using an input device, such as a stylus. This type of technology is frequently used in health care and the restaurant industry because it is less expensive to produce. They are also highly resistant to liquids and contamination; however, because they comprise soft layers, they are susceptible to damage from sharp implements. If you use some sort of tablet or PalmPilot in your patient care, it is likely a resistive screen on the device that you are using.

TECH TIP

A stylus is an input device that is often used for tablets, computers, or smartphones. These are usually shaped like pens and can be used for writing, tapping, or performing other functions.

There are different types of styli depending on the type of input your screen has:

Digitizer Stylus—This works by using an electrical charge that interacts with a certain type of screen. These styli typically have fine-point, hard tips that are more precise than other options and are therefore the most expensive.

Capacitive Stylus—This works by transferring the conductivity of the human hand to the tip of the stylus. These styli typically have round, soft tips; are some of the least precise styli; and are mid-range in price.

Resistive Stylus—This works by pinpointing pressure in a precise location on the screen to push electrically charged surfaces together, creating a touch point. These styli typically have fine, hard tips; are mid-range in their precision; and are the least expensive to purchase.

The $49 eBay special tablet likely features a resistive touch screen. Although this does not mean that you cannot have an enjoyable experience with this device because of the pressure it requires and its lack of multitouch functions, you may not find it as comfortable to manipulate as devices like the Kindle Fire and Apple iPad, which both feature capacitive screens. If you're looking for a device that will "just work" and allow you to destress after a tough shift, you want a tablet with a little more performance capability.

CAPACITIVE SCREENS

A capacitive touch screen is one that requires minimal touch and is activated by technology that interprets human touch specifically. Depending on your device and the application you are using, a capacitive screen can be single or multitouch. This means that it may respond to only one touch or to many on the screen. Having a multitouch capacitive screen is useful when playing games and manipulating photos. The pinch-to-shrink feature of the iPhone and iPad is an example of a multitouch capability and a gesture recognized by many tablet devices. It senses both of your fingers on the screen at the same time and responds accordingly, zooming a picture in if you spread your fingers out and shrinking the picture if you bring your fingers closer together. This capability could be really helpful if you are reading a nursing article with a really tiny font and want to look at things up close.

Capacitive screens are a newer form of technology and are typically found in more cutting-edge devices. This type of screen is what you see on iPhones and iPads as well as on most major smartphones and tablets. The devices that include this type of screen are usually more responsive and user friendly. With all the advantages of the capacitive screen, and because the technology is newer, the devices that feature them typically carry a higher price point.

Newer Panasonic Toughbook tablets, which are used in many health care settings, feature capacitive touch screens with multitouch gestures. They are much more heavy-duty than something like an iPad and have the ability to run the Windows OS, which many EMRs require.

TECH TIP

Many capacitive screens respond to multitouch gestures. The following are some examples of the multitouch gestures that Apple devices recognize:

Single Finger Tap: This is like clicking a mouse. It is your primary interaction.

Single Finger Flick: Using a single finger, you can flick up or down on the screen to scroll content.

Single Finger Swipe: This move allows you to navigate through content or interact with apps in various ways.

Single Finger Double Tap: This brings an image back to its standard size or zooms in really close very quickly.

Single Finger Touch and Hold: You can highlight text with this method and enable various types of editing functionality.

Shaking the Device: This lets you undo or redo an action.

Two-Finger Pinch: Use two fingers on images and web pages to zoom in and out.

Five-Finger Pinch: If you use your entire hand to grab the screen, then you can close an app and go back to the home page.

Four-Finger Swipe Up: This gestures enables the multitasking bar and gives you a view of the apps you have used recently. This is helpful to quickly switch between the apps you use frequently.

Four-Finger Swipe Left/Right: This gesture allows you to slide one app off the screen and move onto the app you were most recently using. This works well if you use the same few apps constantly (Apple, 2013).

SMART DESIGN AND INTUITIVE INTERFACE

The beauty of almost all tablets is the simplicity of their interface. Most tablets have a minimal number of buttons and feature clean designs. This is actually really great for the user, because it means there are far fewer buttons to learn and be aware of. This also means there are fewer parts to break. Most tablets include a few standard features in their designs, such as a power switch, volume buttons, headphone jack, and speakers. There may or may not be a screen-orientation lock (which keeps your screen in one position even if you rotate the device). Most non-Apple devices also feature a way to add additional storage to your tablet via an external memory card.

The reason why many nurses get annoyed with technology is because it can be overly complicated. Tablets eliminate some of the muss and fuss from getting things done. The tablet market is very competitive, and most manufacturers attempt to make devices as easy to use as possible. This might mean decreasing the number of taps needed to get something done or allowing users to customize the device to fit their needs.

The hardware and OS of the tablet are very important, but you shouldn't forget to think about the actual apps you are going to be doing your work on. If you are documenting on an EMR, it is important that this app be designed to be used on a tablet and isn't just a secondary functionality. A smart software developer customizes software to fit the device and doesn't just offer loose adaptations that happen to be available for a tablet.

TECH TIP

If you are involved in selecting devices or software for hospital implementation, you need to be realistic about what you expect nurses to do with it. If you are annoyed or frustrated with how something works, chances are high that staff nurses will be as well.

BATTERY LIFE AND STANDBY

One of a tablet's most attractive features is its ability to awaken and be used almost instantly. Your tablet device stays on and in standby mode in a much more responsive manner than a traditional computer. The battery life is also considerably longer than that of any laptop you've ever owned. Average battery life on a tablet ranges anywhere from 6 to 10 hours, while standby time (how long your battery lasts when the tablet is not in use) is up to 30 days. This means that unless you use your device heavily, you do not have to be worried about charging your device every day to ensure that you'll be able to use it. With casual use, you can go several days or even a week in between charges. However, you'll likely fall in love with your tablet and use it frequently, so you'll want to charge it often. You can get a car charger or an extra wall charger fairly inexpensively, so in my opinion, this is really a nonissue.

If you're working an 8- to 12-hour day, then you need a battery that will last. Who has time to sit and take a breather while your tablet recharges? Most nurses would agree, "Ain't nobody got time for that." Some tablets offer the ability to hot swap a battery without even turning the device off. Little extras like this can really help a nurse out.

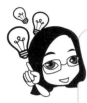

TECH TIP

Hot swapping a battery is a nice innovation if you have a device that is heavily used with little time available for charging. Nurses who work on the floor and share a device with others have the potential to run into this scenario often. This type of device allows you to swap out your battery while the device is still powered on. This is really handy, because you won't lose what you are doing if you need to switch out your battery.

STORAGE CAPACITY AND ENCRYPTION

The amount of available storage on a tablet is far less than that of a traditional computer, because the hard drives are kept in a smaller location, and the tinier the hardware, the more expensive it is to produce. Most tablets include anywhere from 4GB to 64GB of storage. For most people, even the minimal amount is plenty for casual use. The amount of storage you need is related to the amount of content you want available on your device at all times. Since the invention of cloud computing (which we discussed when we talked about Google Drive in Chapter 2), most people find it less necessary to have all their music, movies, or photos available at any given time. What you should consider for storage purposes is the number of apps you are going to download and use frequently.

If you are using a work-provided tablet that patient information will be stored on, it is important that the device be encrypted. This ensures that even if the device is lost or stolen, criminals will not be able to retrieve the data. The friendly folks in your IT department should take care of the encryption process for you. If you are not sure whether your device is encrypted or whether it should be, you can always ask. If you have inquired about the safety of patient data but don't feel as though you are getting adequate answers from your IT department, you can always involve compliance and your medical records department.

CODE CAUTION

It's a big deal if a tablet with PHI is lost or stolen and the device is not encrypted. This is a HIPAA breach and comes with costly penalties and increased scrutiny for your organization. Don't think twice—encrypt your device!

OPERATING SYSTEMS

You likely are already familiar with some form of computer OS; this is the structure, file system, and interface that allows you to "do things" on your computer. It's what makes the computer boot up, run applications to access the Internet, and run the EMR system that your health care organization uses to document patient care. Because most health care organizations have either switched to or are in the process of switching to electronic charting, you likely already have some experience working with a computer OS.

If you use a computer at home, it most likely runs one of the two most popular operating systems: Microsoft's Windows or Apple's Mac OS. If you have a computer at home that runs anything other than these two, then you are far too nerdy to need this guide!

Tablets also have different operating systems, depending on their manufacturers. The three dominant operating systems are Apple's iOS, Google's Android, and Microsoft's Windows. Each OS offers a unique experience for the consumer, and each differs in the number of types of apps (applications/software) that they can support.

TECH TIP

Many EMRs only run on Windows-based systems. Check with your software manufacturer to determine what your options are.

iOS

The Apple iPad is without question the most popular tablet. Even at its $499 starting price tag, it outsells the others and has the most passionate fans. The reason for this is likely in the simplicity of the iOS operating system as well as the more than 900,000 screened apps available in the iTunes store. The iOS operating system has been designed so that anyone can easily pick up the device and in a matter of moments use it meaningfully. Ah, meaningful use . . . if that's not a buzzword you hear floating around the hallways of your workplace, chances are it will be in the near future. The term is used in a different context in this manner, but the principles remain the same. Technology should be used meaningfully, easily, and with purpose.

Give an iPad to a toddler, and chances are that child will be able to use it in a matter of moments. If that doesn't demonstrate its simplicity, then what could?

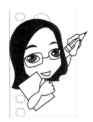

NERDY NOTE

Nurses really need simplicity anywhere we can get it!

The operating system also has many useful apps and tools already integrated. Getting things to work on an iPad is very easy. However, not many EMRs run on iOS. However, a ton of awesome nursing and medical apps can help you provide better patient care.

The simplicity of iOS lends to its intuitiveness. What exactly does it mean when we call a piece of technology intuitive? It means that it has a pretty good idea of how the human brain works and how a typical user is going to interact with a device. Basically, it knows what you are going to do before you do. This eliminates much of the thought needed to use a tablet, and more specifically an iPad, because most everything "just works."

If a child can pick it up and figure it out in a matter of minutes, you can certainly do the same. You are a nurse, after all, and that's no small accomplishment!

iOS is also a very secure operating system that does not get viruses or malware. The apps that you can download are screened and tested prior to being released to iTunes, which also helps maintain the security of the iPad and helps ensure a better experience overall with the apps that you download and use. In health care, it's imperative that environments involving patient data be very secure and have very stable operating systems. iOS offers this in an environment that is user-friendly to many nurses.

CODE CAUTION

If you use your iPad for your work email, then there are chances that PHI might come through your email. Make sure that you are clear on your employer's policies regarding work email on personal devices and that these devices are secure.

ANDROID

Android is the OS that most tablets (other than the iPad, of course) base their interface on. However, what you see and experience with one device may not always look the same on another tablet. For example, a Kindle Fire has an Android-based OS, but its interface looks nothing like the version of Android that a Google Nexus tablet features. The version of Android your tablet has also influences which apps marketplace you have access to. On many

Android-based tablets, including the Kindle Fire, you may not have the ability to access the entire Android marketplace. This is because it uses an Android skeleton for its OS rather than the full versions seen on other devices, like the Google Nexus.

Android tablets are not often used directly in the health care setting to document patient care, but they are often used by nurses to help them deliver better care. Many nursing and health care apps can be used on an Android tablet to help you with lab values, diseases, and medications. The limited apps market is not really a problem for most casual tablet users. The most popular apps, and the ones you will likely find to be the most valuable, will usually be available in the apps store. The exception to this rule may be relevant nursing and medical apps. You will likely find these lacking in the devices that offer access to anything less than a full Android marketplace.

Android Is Open Source   Android is an open-source OS. *The Android Open Source Project* is led by Google. Being "open source" means that it is possible to take the skeleton of the Android OS and manipulate it to fit a product. This is why you will find Android on multiple devices made by multiple companies, but it also leads to a different experience on different tablets. You may already be familiar with a version of the Android OS if you use a non-Apple smartphone. If you already own an Android-based smartphone, then you'd likely find that using an Android-based tablet would be very similar.

Not All Androids Are Created Equal   When comparing tablets with the Android OS, it is important to know that not all Android OS tablets are created equal. Not only may the hardware of a tablet vary, but the build of the OS will often be a custom version for that particular device. This is in comparison to iOS, which looks and functions the same on any iPad you use (assuming, of course, it has been updated to the most current version).

Google Play Store   If you are looking for an Android tablet that you can access helpful nursing apps with, then you will need to make sure you have a device that has the ability to access the full Google Play Store. This will give you many more options in nursing and medical apps.

It is relevant to mention that the full Android marketplace often has unscreened content and therefore has the potential for malware and viruses that can infect your tablet. So having a Kindle Fire that limits your access to the full marketplace is not really a problem in the grand scheme of things. If anything, this keeps you safe from yourself and prevents you from breaking your shiny gadget.

Although the primary difference in the Android and iOS operating systems is their app stores, the functionality is somewhat different. Android offers a greater ability to customize and alter your experience, but Android is the younger OS, and some of its applications do not appear as polished as their iOS counterparts.

MICROSOFT'S WINDOWS

Windows 8 and Windows RT are the tablet offerings form Microsoft. Windows 8 is the same OS that is used on desktop systems, which usually means that most EMR systems can run on these devices. Windows RT tablets are app-based devices with far fewer app choices available, which pretty much guarantees that you aren't going to be able to run an EMR on it and that your nursing app choices are going to be very limited.

Microsoft has struggled to create a user interface that works on a tablet but is also a workhorse. Some tech experts believe that Microsoft has finally accomplished this with Windows 8, but many aren't convinced. I personally think that Windows 8 is a strong competitor in the tablet market and is the only OS that health care organizations can practically use.

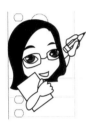

NERDY NOTE
If you're using a tablet for work, it's probably Windows based.

APPS

One of the defining differences between using a computer and using a tablet is how apps (short for applications) work. A good app is one that is designed from the ground up to be interacted with as effortlessly as possible with the understanding that you'll be using a series of gestures involving one or more fingers to manipulate it.

More than 900,000 apps are available in the iTunes store alone, and the Android market is rapidly catching up.

Some examples of specific apps and categories of apps that you might find useful include the following:

+ Games: Angry Birds, Words With Friends, Farmville

+ Financial: Mint, Check, bank-specific software, budget-planning tools

+ Education and Reading: GoodReader, multiple ebook apps

+ Productivity: word processors, planning and to-do lists

+ Music services: Pandora, Sirius XM

✛ Video content: YouTube, Netflix, Hulu

✛ Social media: Facebook, Twitter, LinkedIn, Google+

✛ Nursing and health care: Epocrates Essentials, MedPage, and Nursing Drug Guide

Having an iOS device gives you access to the iTunes Apps Store. The iTunes store has a screening process that helps filter out undesirable applications as well as ensure the security of iOS users. This is the primary reason why iOS devices do not get viruses and other forms of malware.

You want access to a wide variety of apps if you want your tablet to help you with nursing-related tasks. Because nursing apps aren't used by the general population of tablet users, these apps might not be reviewed by certain device manufacturers for a while if ever. Having a device that gives you access to all apps in the Google Play Store allows you to decide which apps you think would be helpful in your career.

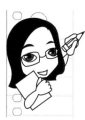

NERDY NOTE

Many apps for nurses are categorized as Medical or Health Apps. Browsing through these sections can be really interesting and informative.

TABLETS MAKE TECHNOLOGY FUN

Although it may seem like owning a tablet could potentially be an overwhelming experience, the reality is that most people who purchase one really enjoy using it. Tablets serve a different purpose from a smartphone or a computer by combining the portability of a smartphone with the screen size and more powerful processing power of a computer. If you have neither of these items, then a tablet is an excellent way to acclimate yourself to some of the new technologies that are available.

Tablets are different from computers and phones, because we don't yet rely on them to function in our daily lives. Because of that, there is much more room to have fun with them.

You work hard taking care of patients and making their lives better. Don't you deserve something just for you that can be fun and useful too? If you like to read books, enjoy and share pictures of your family, watch TV or movies, or surf the Internet at all, then you'd enjoy owning a tablet.

PROTECTING AND ACCESSORIZING YOUR TABLET

Whether you use a tablet for work or play, you'll want to invest in a few accessories to make your tablet-owning experience more pleasurable:

✦ Case or sleeve

✦ Extra wall charger

✦ Car charger

✦ Screen protector

✦ Stylus

✦ Bluetooth speakers

✦ Charging dock or portable power blocks

✦ Dock or stand

✦ Headphones (traditional wired or wireless Bluetooth)

✦ Bluetooth keyboard

Every day, more and more accessories are being created to accompany your tablet device. Once you start exploring the possibilities for tablet accessories, it becomes almost like exploring possibilities in nursing specialties—you can just get sucked into the vastness of it all. You'll find items you love and hate and items that you cannot understand why anyone would want to own. But, just like with nursing specialties, there is something just right for everyone. And what is right for you today doesn't have to be what is right for you tomorrow—you always have the option to switch things up. It's a wonderful luxury afforded to nurses in their professional choices and in their tablet accessory choices.

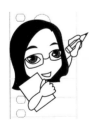

NERDY NOTE
Nursing is a career where you should never be bored. Technology is the same way. There is always something new to learn and a new area of interest that you can explore further to become an expert on.

Regardless of which tablet you choose to call your very own, you are going to want to make sure you get something to protect it. A case can vary in form and function and range from as little as $10 to more than $100. You can even order customizable skins for your tablet that feature your favorite football team's mascot or pictures of your kids. Of course, you can opt for a traditional leather style or hard plastic case off the shelf as well. Some cases even incorporate Bluetooth keyboards, which can transform your tablet experience into something entirely different all together.

Many charging docks and speaker systems are also available to enhance your tablet experience. There are even accessories like digital scales and pedometers that can link with your tablet via Bluetooth. Every day, new accessories are added that can expand the possibilities of tablet computing.

HOW NURSES CAN USE TABLETS

Aside from the ability to connect you to social networking and other various leisure activities, tablets can also have value in your professional life. Tablets make it easier to access information, expand your nursing knowledge, and stay up to date on emerging trends in health care. They can also allow you to quickly access lab values and information about diseases, medication contraindications, and more information than you can even imagine that can help you deliver better patient care.

You can use a tablet to easily stay up to date on evidence-based practice to improve your patient care. Open apps on your tablet to learn more about a patient's medical conditions, look up information about medications via a drug guide, or find guides and videos related to various nursing procedures.

Depending on the policies of your health care organization, you can use a tablet to enhance your patient care in many different ways. But before you start using a tablet on the floor, you should always check your employer's policies regarding specific devices. If they are generic, you should always ask for clarification.

CODE CAUTION

Don't make assumptions about which types of technology are OK on the floor. Be proactive and ask about policies. If you are in charge of making policies, be sure that a policy on tablets in the workplace exists. And "no tablets allowed" should not be part of it!

One of the biggest ways you can utilize a tablet is to educate yourself and your patients. You can read nursing articles and keep yourself up to date on the latest evidence-based practices. You can also use tablets to share hospital-approved videos, images, and other educational materials with your patients.

It should be noted that this area is newly emerging, and many health care organizations have not fully embraced all the value that can come with fully utilizing technology for care providers. It is up to you as a patient advocate to ensure that you supporting the use of this technology. Doing so can and will help improve the care you provide as well as show your patients that you and your health care organization are focused on providing technologically advanced medical care.

There is a very real reason why hospitals are moving away from paper: Digital tools and technology are enhancing the care we are able to provide in more ways than we ever imagined. Tablets are just one of those ways.

WHAT DOCTORS ARE ALREADY DOING WITH TABLETS

Many physicians are already utilizing tablets to enhance the patient care they provide. Applications for viewing EMRs, cardiac strips, fetal monitoring, and more are being utilized by the medical community. Depending on how technology-focused your health care organization is, you may or may not have noticed an increase in tablet use.

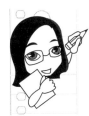

NERDY NOTE
Why should doctors be the only ones who get to use cutting-edge technology to improve patient care?

Physicians can also use tablets to involve patients more directly in their care. They can pull up patient scans and other data and educate the patients on their conditions right at the bedside. They can also use apps that show basic anatomy to describe surgical procedures and help patients better understand the care they are going to receive.

Tablets also afford physicians with easier access to updates on pertinent health care information. They can read journals regarding changes in medical standards if they are easily available on their tablets. They are also able to remotely access patient records while on the go and make better assessments of situations while they are on call.

THE POSSIBILITIES FOR TABLETS IN PATIENT EDUCATION AND FOLLOW-UP CARE

One of the largest responsibilities of any nurse's role in providing patient care is to educate the patient. Much of this education comes in the form of printed documents and paperwork that a patient may not ever look at. It's a wasteful, outdated way to deliver education to patients.

Imagine if instead of providing your patient with a folder of paper, you could hand the person a tablet that came loaded with all the education needed. It could display videos, pictures, articles, links to relevant and helpful websites, the patient's discharge paperwork, information about the patient's medications, and a wealth of other resources. The next time the patient came in for a visit, he or she could present you with the tablet, and, with a few touches, you could easily update the device with any additional information or changes that are relevant to the patient's condition.

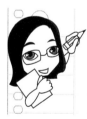

NERDY NOTE
A hospital system could easily manage tablet education for a controlled population, and there are possibly even grants to subsidize the cost.

Now, of course, the decision to utilize technology like this is entirely up to your hospital administrators, but it is up to you to advocate for these advances. Don't be the nurse crossing your arms in the corner saying, "I can't" or "I won't" or "I remember when we didn't have to do all this!" Be the nurse standing up front, eager and excited about the improvements that new technology will provide for your patient care. You'll find not only that you are better able to handle the changes associated with emerging new technologies but that you enjoy being a nurse more. You enjoy utilizing computer charting. You enjoy sharing with patients the advances in their health care that are made possible by technology. Your patients will be impressed with your care and give your health care organization higher ratings, which will lead to increases in pay for performance and, I hope, eventual increases in your own salary as well.

Be an early adopter. Your seniors and superiors will notice your desire and ability to embrace change and innovation, and opportunities will start lining up for you. Technology, computers, and electronic documentation are only going become more integral to your nursing care. It's high time you step up to learn the value of it.

HOW PATIENTS CAN USE TABLETS TO IMPROVE THEIR HEALTH CARE

Tablets put valuable information in patients' hands. Apps can help remind patients to take their medications, track their blood glucose levels, and find recipes to improve their diets. The touch screen allows those who may have difficulty using a traditional mouse access to the same information that others have online.

Tons of recipe and dietary apps are available. If an individual only used an iPad to improve eating habits, it would be money well spent. The money saved in health care–related costs due to comorbidities acquired from a poor diet would easily cover the $499 cost of the device. Luckily, an iPad acts as a whole lot more than just the world's largest cookbook.

TECH TIP

The key to getting patients to use technology as a way to improve their health is to teach them how. Ask your patients whether they have tablets. Regardless of their answers, you can tell them about helpful resources that are available in the form of apps and websites.

Fitness apps can help you plan workouts and stay on track with your diet. Many apps let you count calories and plan meals. Apps let you manipulate your own image to see what you might look like if you put on a few hundred pounds. If a digitized image of yourself several hundred pounds overweight isn't enough to inspire you to get fit, then not much will.

With new Bluetooth health accessories like scales, blood pressure cuffs, and Fitbits, patients can track their overall health wirelessly. The technology even exists today to transmit this information to their physicians without their intervention if they so choose. It is only a matter of years before this practice becomes commonplace.

NERDY NOTE

A Fitbit is a personal fitness device that can help you keep track of how your body responds to daily activity and exercise. These small devices make contact with your skin by clipping on a shirt or pants or being worn as a bracelet and then measuring your pulse and other key health indicators. Many people consider them to be glorified pedometers, but they can be really useful in helping you understand the level of activity you actually perform each day. For best results, most users couple the Fitbit with its smartphone app to help them manage their overall health and stay commited to living a healthier lifestyle.

Although Fitbit is the most popular gadget of this sorts, many similar options are available, including Nike+ FuelBand, Jawbone UP, and BodyMedia FIT. If you're looking for something that will help you stay motivated to be healthier without the expense of a personal trainer, these gizmos might be the next best thing.

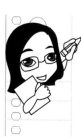

NERDY NOTE

Wireless health devices may soon be something that we are all using. Imagine if all your health information were automatically logged each morning and then sent to your physician. The technology exists today—it's just a matter of implementing it in a useful and practical way.

IMPROVEMENTS IN THE PATIENT EXPERIENCE

Pretty soon, tablets will be so commonplace you will see more people sitting in a physician's office holding a tablet than a magazine. A patient will be handed one upon arriving at a physician's office and use it to complete the standard health questions that have been traditionally filled out on paper. All the information will be wirelessly transmitted to the computer system and become part of the patient's medical record.

Later, a patient can use a tablet or computer at home to access an online patient portal. This information will include the results from the labs the patient had drawn and allow the patient to schedule follow-up appointments with physicians, access a list of all current medications, and even pay the bill. The patient will have access to all medical information in one location without having to fill out forms, pay a fee, or request the paperwork from a specific office.

WHAT DID YOU LEARN ABOUT TABLETS?

This chapter should have been really fun. Why? Because I'm fun, and tablets are fun, and when the two come together, it's guaranteed to be more fun than a barrel of monkeys. Even with all this fun to distract you, I hope you paid attention, because I've got questions and you've got answers:

+ Which operating system are most EMR systems designed to work on?

+ How can you use a tablet to improve nursing care?

+ What is encryption, and why is it important in health care?

Six chapters down, and three to go. You feel like a bona fide nerd yet?

REFERENCE

Apple. (2013, May 1). Platform characteristics. *iOS Developer Library*. Retrieved from http://developer.apple.com/library/ios/#documentation/userexperience/conceptual/mobilehig/Characteristics/Characteristics.html

7

ELECTRONIC DOCUMENTATION: EHR, EMR, PHR, AND OTHER DIGITAL DOCUMENTATION

Meaningful Use and other government-driven initiatives have led to a surge in health care organizations' adoptions of electronic medical records (EMRs). Many nurses feel greatly inconvenienced by being forced to adapt to EMRs and believe that the time it takes to access and document in them takes valuable time away from delivering good patient care. Patients are typically accepting of the use of EMRs but often do not understand how this system can improve their care.

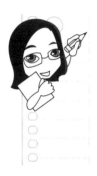

NERDY NOTE

One of the best pieces of education you can give to patients is how the EMRs make their care better. I really like using the example of bedside medication verification. The bracelets, barcodes, and scanning combine with a sophisticated EMR component that helps ensure that the patient gets the right medication. Although many patients understand the basics of EMRs, they really appreciate it when you give them concrete examples of how these systems improve their care.

Although change is always difficult, there is little doubt that health care is constantly changing for the positive. If you want to give your patients the best care possible, you need to meet the most current standards. EMRs greatly improve access to pertinent patient care information and in the long run can even improve patient outcomes.

As nurses, we must make sure that we are comfortable and familiar with new technologies used to deliver patient care. We must also ensure that we take the time to educate patients on all the benefits that electronic records offer. The last thing a patient needs to hear is that you don't know how to use the EMR or that you hate using a computer. This can greatly decrease the patient's confidence level in your abilities and cause undue stress.

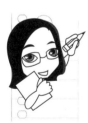

NERDY NOTE

The few moments you spend explaining the EMR system will likely save you time overall. If a patient understands why you are "playing on the computer over there," the person is more likely to let you complete your documentation.

THE BITTERSWEET GOOD-BYE TO THE PAPER CHART

I've encountered many nurses in my career who have mourned the loss of their paper charts. They speak of paper records fondly as if they were old friends from college whom they lost touch with. Their longing for the return of their beloved paper charts can almost be equated to the mourning of a lost loved one. To many nurses, being forced to convert paper charts to EMRs is a tragedy. If only they could find their paper charts on Facebook! At least then they could pretend they were still friends.

I can't even imagine how high a stack of paper charts would be if it contained the amount of documentation that we track today. Paper may have worked in the past, but we were also keeping track of and submitting far less data than we are today.

Converting to an EMR can be painful, to say the least. Many processes that formerly required only checkmarks on a page now necessitate several mouse clicks. Nurses get annoyed when processes that were once simple are made overly complicated. In reality, we should have been converting to EMRs incrementally, perfecting pieces and adding new functionality as technology improved. But that's just not the way change usually happens.

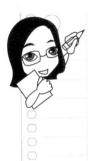

NERDY NOTE

You can take several approaches to implementing EMRs. Most organizations choose to do this all at once, because it tends to prevent push-back. If everyone is on the same page, then you don't have the same number of stragglers that you would if you incorporated just one a piece at a time. Although I wish rolling new initiatives out slowly was a real option, unfortunately some health care workers make this nearly impossible.

Usually the news of an EMR is sprung on you suddenly, and implementation is all or nothing. Nurses and other members of the health care team are flung into the deep end, left wondering whether they will sink or swim. They drown in the new way of doing things and often feel helpless and overwhelmed. There isn't enough support in the world to make such a massive change completely painless, but I know that many organizations could do a much better job in preparing their employees to use EMRs. On the other hand, with proper planning and the right resources, some organizations do a great job of implementing EMRs. I believe that if positive attitudes, clear communication, transparency, and requests for feedback are utilized, this type of project can be much more successful. One of the worst things about working on the night shift as a nurse is that you hardly ever hear anything from the horse's mouth. You hear news of changes and expectations through the grapevine and often have so many added opinions by the time you receive the information that it's hard to formulate your own. If health care organizations want nurses to embrace change and EMRs more positively, then they need to communicate with all nurses directly. They need to be transparent and always ask for feedback. Most importantly, anyone in a leadership role (even a charge nurse) should approach change in a positive manner (even if the person secretly really hates it).

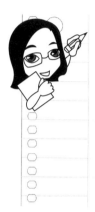

NERDY NOTE

Many people look to others to gauge their reactions to a change and often form their opinions based at least partially on this information. If everything they hear about EMRs is negative, then the implementation is probably going to be a negative experience for them, regardless of how the experience could turn out. Most nurses are leaders in some regard and have someone to whom they delegate responsibilities. In this leadership role, we need to be aware of how our actions and opinions can negatively affect those around us. This is especially true when implementing change, but it's also just a good attitude to maintain in general.

WHY YOU HAVE TO CLICK SO MANY BOXES

A couple of the most frequently asked questions that nurses ask are "Why does it take so many clicks to get to the screen I need?" and "Why do I have to check so many boxes?"

Answering the first question is a little easier than the second. Part of the answer is simply because we're still learning how to use EMRs. We don't have the system streamlined yet. We haven't figured out how to eliminate all the redundancy. Unfortunately, we're really in the infancy of the technology. We're learning every day, and eventually things will improve, but it's a two steps forward and one step back process: Every time we fix two things, it seems like something else breaks. In many IT departments, a large portion of the staff's time is spent putting out fires, which leaves little time for improving existing systems and processes.

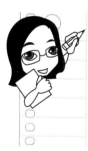

NERDY NOTE

With the proper amount of planning, budgeting, and staff, the number of fires that have to be put out can be greatly reduced. Many hospitals see the IT department as a service center rather than a key player in the business. For this situation to improve, IT needs to be taken seriously and involved from the beginning in any projects that will require their help.

With all the advances in televisions, cars, and computers, it seems a little bit silly that health care technology is lagging so far behind. It's really kind of pathetic to think that the technology that many of us carry in our pockets is more cutting edge than what those in the medical industry have access to.

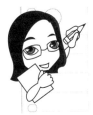

NERDY NOTE

Hospitals don't like to spend money on technology. It's expensive, and many people who make major purchasing decisions like to spend as little as possible. Innovation in health care is often stifled by the all-mighty budget.

EMRs are often designed with continuity of care in mind. They should allow a patient's data to be accessible in many areas and to many different clinicians. However, the software also needs the ability to define who can and can't access this data. This sometimes increases the number of menus that have to be clicked to get to the intervention or assessment that you are looking for.

CODE CAUTION

Patient charts are on a "need-to-know" basis. If you have no good reason to be in a chart, do yourself a favor and stay out of it. Not doing so could be a HIPAA violation and result in disciplinary action, termination, or even a costly fine.

But perk up, dear friend! I promise you that the clicking will be reduced. As time progresses and workflows become more refined, you will start to notice that accessing the functions you need in an EMR will become less complicated.

That brings me to the second question: "Why do I have to check so many boxes?" This question has many answers. The first and most important reason is that old saying we all know and adore: "If you didn't document it, it wasn't done." But what many may not realize is that another quotation goes hand in hand with documentation: "If you can't find it, it doesn't exist." Simply writing down the information isn't always good enough. This is the very reason that the narrative nursing note is going the way of the dinosaur.

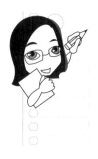

NERDY NOTE

I'm a little old-school when it comes to certain aspects of nursing. I would happily wear whites and a cap if it wouldn't get me laughed off the nursing unit. A well-crafted nursing note should be considered an art form, almost like poetry. And as much as I love electronic documentation, I am sometimes saddened by the fact that a narrative nurse's note is now hardly ever utilized.

You are required to check boxes, pull down answer choices, and select predefined responses in interventions and assessments because these data can later be retrieved and measured to determine whether we are meeting key areas of public health. This information can tell us how many patients are smokers and how many had a positive TB skin test. Simply writing a narrative note about these assessment findings is not good enough. This type of data cannot be reported, and it's difficult to quickly find relevant information in a patient's chart.

Have you ever sat down and attempted to quickly get an idea of the general health of a patient by reading just the nurse's narrative notes? If they are handwritten, you are going to have a hard enough time deciphering them. Then you need to be able to spend fewer than 5 minutes on the chart to find relevant information to care for the individual. It can be nearly impossible. Key items get missed, and the concept of continuity of care is just completely shattered. EMRs and Meaningful Use will eventually change all that.

DIFFERENCES AMONG EMRS, EHRS, AND PHRS

Many people do not realize there are differences among an electronic medical record (EMR), an electronic health record (EHR), and a personal health record (PHR). I myself am guilty of often using the terms "EHR" and "EMR" interchangeably. However, some defining differences distinguish these health and medical records.

Wikipedia (2013) has this to say about the topic:

> The terms EHR, EPR (electronic patient record), and EMR (electronic medical record) are often used interchangeably, although differences between them can be defined. The EMR can, for example, be defined as the patient record created in hospitals and ambulatory environments, which can serve as a data source for the EHR. It is important to note that an EHR is generated and maintained within an institution,

such as a hospital, integrated delivery network, clinic, or physician office, to give patients, physicians and other health care providers, employers, and payers or insurers access to a patient's medical records across facilities.

A personal health record (PHR) is, in modern parlance, generally defined as an EHR that the individual patient controls. (Electronic health record, 2013, para. 3)

ELECTRONIC MEDICAL RECORD

Wikipedia says:

> An electronic medical record (EMR) is a computerized medical record created in an organization that delivers care, such as a hospital or physician's office. Electronic medical records tend to be a part of a local stand-alone health information system that allows storage, retrieval, and modification of records. (Electronic medical record, 2013, para. 1)

An EMR (or electronic medical patient record) is the collective term for the chart and all documentation recorded while taking care of a patient. In hospitals that have completely converted to EMRs, these records will be the location for pretty much all the data related to a patient's care and are to be viewed by health care staff on an as-needed-only basis. The purpose of EMRs is to document care provided and communicate orders, results, and other values to any health care provider who requires the information while caring for a patient. These data are protected by HIPAA laws, and access is limited to only the staff caring for the patient.

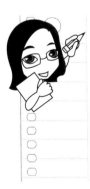

NERDY NOTE

Although HIPAA is sometimes shoved directly down our throats, and just hearing the term is enough to make an eye twitch, this law actually does good things. It forces health care organizations to be accountable with patient information. Think about patient records as if they were your own. Would you want everyone and their mamas seeing your lab results, peeping at your address, or taking a glance at your Social Security number? Patients trust us at a time when they are most vulnerable. We need to make sure we always respect that, and HIPAA helps us do this.

Patients do not have direct access to their EMRs during their hospitalization. However, they can request copies of their records, and health care organizations have to comply with these demands in a reasonable manner. Depending on the stage of Meaningful Use that a hospital is in, this information must be delivered to the patients electronically.

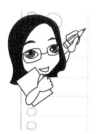

NERDY NOTE

The choice of electronic formats can be slightly subjective. In some cases, this might mean putting information onto a CD or jump drive. Ultimately, patients should be able to access their own medical records on demand via a Health Information Exchange (HIE).

Many EMR vendors create and support EMR systems that aid in the delivery of patient care in the acute, long term, ambulatory, and home care settings (just to name a few).

ELECTRONIC HEALTH RECORD

Wikipedia says:

> An electronic health record (EHR) is an evolving concept defined as a systematic collection of electronic health information about individual patients or populations. It is a record in digital format that is theoretically capable of being shared across different health care settings. In some cases, this sharing can occur by way of network-connected, enterprise-wide information systems and other information networks or exchanges. EHRs may include a range of data, including demographics, medical history, medication and allergies, immunization status, laboratory test results, radiology images, vital signs, personal stats like age and weight, and billing information. (Electronic health record, 2013, para. 1)

An EHR (or electronic health care record) is a record of information from health care providers and organizations that a patient can access at leisure via an online location. This concept works in theory, but because of the many different programming languages that exist, EMRs and EHRs don't always play nicely with each other, although this situation is improving drastically. With the Meaningful Use or ARRA initiative, hospitals and other health care organizations are going to have to meet patients' needs for easy access to their medical records by providing those patients with patient portals, which will be EHRs that contain all your health information from one health care system.

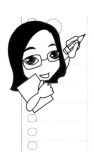

NERDY NOTE

The Health Information Technology for Economic and Clinical Health (HITECH) Act, as part of the American Recovery and Reinvestment Act (ARRA), which was signed into law in 2009 (ARRA Meaningful Use snapshot), establishes Meaningful Use criteria, an EMR adoption incentive program, and ultimately monetary penalties for health care organizations that do not adopt electronic documentation standards.

PERSONAL HEALTH RECORD

Wikipedia says:

> A personal health record, or PHR, is a health record where health data and information related to the care of a patient is maintained by the patient. This stands in contrast with the more widely used electronic medical record, which is operated by institutions (such as a hospital) and contains data entered by clinicians or billing data to support insurance claims. The intention of a PHR is to provide a complete and accurate summary of an individual's medical history that is accessible online. The health data on a PHR might include patient-reported outcome data, lab results, data from devices such as wireless electronic weighing scales or collected passively from a smartphone. (Personal health record, 2013, para. 1)

Basically this is a record of personal health that the patient maintains. These are great tools to help improve care across the continuum and really can empower patients to take responsibility for their own well-being and overall health. Northern Illinois Physicians for Connectivity (2009) published an article that states, "The potential value of this secure electronic exchange and sharing of confidentially protected information can be both cost and time efficient and increase compliance in managing acute or chronic conditions and/or health maintenance activities to stay on track with preventive health programs."

Several companies offer these PHRs in both paid and free versions. Microsoft HealthVault is one of the most popular. However, PHRs are very one-sided. The patient is completely responsible for keeping all information up to date, often by manually typing this information into a database.

PHRs are often being absorbed into EHRs to offer patients a much more practical and dynamic health record. These systems allow patients to access their health data, provide direct communication with health care providers, and in most cases add their own documentation.

Because this record can be updated by health care providers and by the patient, it offers the best of both worlds. The type of system available to you depends on the health care system in which the patient receives care.

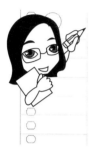

NERDY NOTE

These EHRs are often segregated by health systems. As time progresses and the time frames for Meaningful Use pass, there will be a greater focus in putting this information into statewide and even national health databases. Although the thought of this is scary for some (especially if the NSA has access to it!), it means that if you are sick or injured, your medical providers will have access to your complete medical history at any given time.

CONTINUITY IS KEY!

For patients to get the best health care possible, it is vital that we work toward the goal of having all forms of health and medical records available electronically. This change is critical for interoperability and necessary so that we can more easily communicate with one another. Patients need to be just as involved in their own health care as those providing that care.

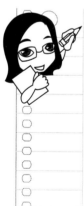

NERDY NOTE

"Interoperability" is a big buzzword in health care IT these days. What this basically means is that systems should talk to each other. Historically, health care records have worked within themselves and sent data to another system built on different computer code, a tedious process involving multiple steps and computer programs. With Meaningful Use, EMR software vendors are stepping up to the plate and making health information accessible in other systems.

This is just one example that demonstrates the importance of nursing informatics. Without having rededicated and passionate nurses in IT, these dreams could not become a reality.

Although many people believe that we are already living in the age of the EMR, some truly wonderful outcomes can and likely will develop as hospitals, other health care organizations, and patients themselves start to get with the electronic program. Personally, I get very excited when I think about all the possibilities that are at our fingertips in health care right now. And I get even more excited about the tools that will be available to both patients and health care providers in the very near future.

NERDY NOTE

According to the American Medical Informatics Association (2009), nursing informatics is the "science and practice [that] integrates nursing, its information and knowledge, with management of information and communication technologies to promote the health of people, families, and communities worldwide." But, I just call it Nerdy Nursing.

As an informatics nurse, I am a bridge for communication between health care and information technology. I speak both nerd and nurse, so I can easily translate the wants and needs of both parties and often play the role of facilitator and mediator. I am also skilled in analytics and have the ability to problem solve and implement process improvements by utilizing technology.

Informatics nurses function in many roles. In some health care originations, their primary role is in education. In my role, I primarily serve as an EMR software analyst and in an educational role when needed.

The need for nurses in health care information technology continues to grow. If you're good with computers, highly adaptable, and passionate about improving patient care, then nursing informatics may be the right career path for you.

MEANINGFUL USE: HOW AND WHY IT MATTERS TO YOU AND YOUR PATIENTS

You've likely heard the buzzwords "Meaningful Use," but it's also entirely possible that you have no idea what it means. There are three stages of Meaningful Use, and each of these stages builds on the other. Information about the stages of Meaningful Use can be found at HealthIT.gov. In the first stage, you collect data; in the second, you share data; and in the third, you use data to improve patient outcomes. This whole process will take place over several years, with the government giving incentives initially for early adopters and penalties later for health care providers who do not conform.

The key component is that health care providers must acquire and use a certified EMR system. Eventually that record will become an EHR, because it will allow a patient to access the data and take charge of the individual's health records. HealthIT.gov (n.d.) lays it all out in its Policymaking, Regulatory, and Strategy section.

Stage 1 requires electronically capturing data in standardized formats, specifically details on key conditions. It also includes recording quality health measures and various types of public health information. The information collected should be used to better coordinate patient care.

Stage 2 involves advanced clinical processes. This is the stage where HIEs become more prominent. A patient's health information should be more easily shareable at this point, thus allowing a patient greater control over the data.

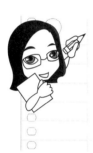

NERDY NOTE

HIEs are web portals where patients' medical records are centrally located. The size and scope of these systems vary but will initially start within health care systems and later expand to statewide and national levels. These systems should contain all the health records for a patient, allowing the patient to interact with health care providers and ultimately improve continuity of care.

Stage 3 is where the *meaningful* aspect comes in. At this point, the data will be used in a meaningful way to improve patient outcomes. Patients will have increased access to tools to help them manage their care. Physicians and other health care providers will have access to comprehensive patient records through robust HIEs. Health care providers will have access to clinical decision support tools. This stage will also include the ability to see trends on conditions and health concerns across the population of the United States.

The goal of Meaningful Use is what makes all this electronic charting more practical and functional. This movement will eventually help patients receive better care with greater consistency. To nurses, it's just a matter of clicking, scrolling, and typing, but to patients, it's the path to better health care.

WOW, THAT WAS MEANINGFUL!

By now you should be able to distinguish between the types of medical and health records, know what Meaningful Use is, and understand the importance of electronic documentation. This was a chapter with a lot of information, so I hope you paid attention:

+ What are the different stages of Meaningful Use?

+ How can patients access their medical records?

+ Why are narrative nursing notes being replaced with check boxes and drop-down menus?

REFERENCES

American Medical Informatics Association. (2009). Working group: Nursing informatics. Retrieved from http://www.amia.org/programs/working-groups/nursing-informatics

ARRA Meaningful Use snapshot. (n.d.). In *Meditech.com*. Retrieved from http://www.meditech.com/Interoperability/flyers/ARRA_snapshot_final.pdf

Electronic health record. (2013, June 7). In *Wikipedia*. Retrieved from http://en.wikipedia.org/wiki/Electronic_health_record

Electronic medical record. (2013, June 12). In *Wikipedia*. Retrieved from http://en.wikipedia.org/wiki/Electronic_medical_record

HealthIT.gov. (n.d.). Policymaking, regulation, & strategy: Meaningful Use. Retrieved from http://www.healthit.gov/policy-researchers-implementers/meaningful-use

Northern Illinois Physicians for Connectivity (NIPFC). (2009). A community view: How personal health records can improve patient care and outcomes in many healthcare settings. *Northern Illinois University*. Retrieved from http://www.niu.edu/rdi/pdf/personal_health_records_and_patient_care_2009.pdf

Personal health record. (2013, June 5). In *Wikipedia*. Retrieved from http://en.wikipedia.org/wiki/Personal_health_record

CAREER ADVANCEMENT AND PROFESSIONAL PRIDE

Good news! Technology can be used to help you advance in your nursing career. You may decide to become an informatics nurse or rely on technology to go back to school to get a higher degree. You can also use technology to educate other nurses in your organization on a new policy, procedure, or patient-centered initiative. Regardless of your purpose, technology can aid your efforts and should be seen as a valuable resource.

In this chapter, I discuss how to use technology and social media to enhance your resume and increase your nursing knowledge. Networking in the digital age can really help improve your career prospects, so I want to make sure you know all about it. I talk about personal branding and what that means for nurses. I then wrap things up by discussing adaptability and flexibility in the nursing workforce.

We discussed informatics nursing in Chapter 7, when we talked about EMR technology. Although many nurses wouldn't dream of leaving the bedside, a career in informatics can be a beautiful thing. It allows you to take care of patients at a different level—touching the lives of hundreds and potentially thousands by ensuring that nurses are better able to do their jobs. By being a translator for nurses in the world of information technology, you ensure that their voices are heard and that nurses aren't made to do extra work or tasks that are inappropriate.

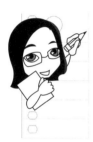

NERDY NOTE

One of the most awesome things I get to do as an informatics nurse is advocate for nurses. I know how it is to work on the floor and feel burdened with the amount of work we have to do. If someone tries to add something to the nursing workload that doesn't make sense, I am the nurse's first line of defense—and I play a good defense.

If you are planning to go back to school for a higher nursing degree, then technology is going to be your best friend. Most schools have at least some of their classes and resources online through complex and interactive communities. This is where you will be able to easily communicate with your instructors and classmates, get class materials, and even participate in group assignments. Before you go back to nursing school, you need to make sure you know your way around a social network, because most schools these days use web-based programs that are very similar.

CODE CAUTION

One thing to consider about the online component to higher education is that you need to be 100% professional. When I was in nursing school, one of my classmates was very inappropriate and suggested on the nursing school–sanctioned forum that I and several others take our heads out of our posteriors (although she said this much more colorfully). This immature and unprofessional behavior resulted in disciplinary action. Although classroom websites are built similarly to Facebook, they aren't a playground and should be used with decorum and professionalism.

If need to educate a large group of nurses, then technology is your friend. You can use video to record your lesson or message and distribute it to large groups of nurses via email. You could also use a website (internal to your organization or external) to write blog entries about different topics that are important or helpful to nurses.

USING SOCIAL MEDIA TO ENHANCE YOUR RESUME

You can use social media to boost your resume in a variety of ways. One way you might be able to beef up your experience is to create content online. Writing a nursing blog or serving as a moderator in an online community is a skill that you should add to your resume. Another idea might be to organize a Twitter chat for nurses.

Some eager nurse entrepreneurs actually run their businesses while relying heavily on technology. I am considered a nurse entrepreneur because I actually make money outside my 9–5 nursing gig by using my nursing skills through my website, freelance writing, and other forms of social media outreach. I know of many other nurses who are doing the very same thing. For some nurses, this type of activity has become their full-time jobs!

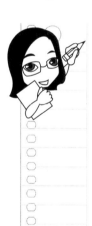

NERDY NOTE

How do you list running a nursing blog on your resume? Easy! You add an entry under your "professional experience" heading that lists your website as the business and describes any activities that you do routinely as part of your blog (but spiff them up so they sound awesome). For example, replying to emails and blog comments might be described as "Added to the online nursing knowledge pool by interacting with nurses on important issues." Creating the content also gets a bullet point on the resume, perhaps something like "Created compelling online content related to important nursing issues and public health concerns." This is blogging, and although it may seem simple, it is actually a huge deal, so give yourself credit for it!

Please note: If you are looking for a quick resume booster, starting up a blog and making a few posts isn't the answer. Your key focus should be content. This doesn't mean you have to update your blog every single day, but you should update the content routinely and post high-quality entries. If potential employers happen to check out your blog, you want them to be impressed by it.

If you want to use social media to enhance your resume, then you need to have a plan. We talked about blogs, Twitter, and forums in Chapter 3. Without a doubt, one of the best ways to add to your resume is to run your own blog, because it gives you a completely new area of work experience to include. It also teaches you valuable skills that will help you be successful online and as a nurse.

Determine whether you want to use blogging and social media solely to boost your resume or whether you actually want to make money doing it. I do both—because I was already putting the work into it, I figured I might as well reap the rewards.

Working on *TheNerdyNurse.com* has really been beneficial to my job in informatics. I have learned a lot about how to manage a database system as well as how to communicate with vendors. Time management, social media etiquette, and marketing know-how are just a few more of the skills that using social media has provided for me.

Blogs run on database management software that files and categorizes all the content you have created. This engine behind the blog enables the pages that appear to be linked together. Although most blog databases work out of the box, if you want to be truly successful, you will need to customize your site a bit. Doing this requires know-how and is yet another skill you can claim on a resume.

TECH TIP

> Luckily, pretty much everything you ever wanted to know about blogging or managing a blogging database (Wordpress or Blogspot) is on Google. If you're lucky, there's even a step-by-step tutorial. So although running a successful blog is hard work and requires you to be open to learning new things, all the resources are at your fingertips after a quick Google search.

As a blogger, you may have opportunities to work with brands and product vendors who want you to review their products or advertise them on your site. Communicating with vendors is a skill that requires professionalism and timeliness, and it does translate to many roles in nursing (management and administration, just to name a few). If your goal is to get a position in one of these areas, then adding this skill to your resume is a must.

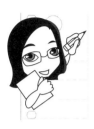

NERDY NOTE

You might ask, "How would I put running a Twitter chat on my resume?" Easy! List it as an accomplishment and word it something like this: "Organized weekly online conversations focusing on various trends and issues in nursing."

Marketing skills may not seem beneficial in nursing, but they most certainly are. The job search alone requires that you be able to sell yourself, and if other nurses have better personal marketing skills, then they are going to have an edge over you. Something as simple as knowing how to present yourself and how to ask for the job may be exactly what sets you apart from the crowd.

Social media and blogging are all about marketing. If you want more followers on Twitter or more visitors to your website, make sure that your product is widely visible and enticing. Marketing via social media, building backlinks through commenting, and participating on forums are all excellent methods to build your online empire—but marketing is also a great skill to have in nursing. If you are competing against other nurses for a job or perhaps other independent contractors as a nurse entrepreneur, it's important that you know how to sell your top product: yourself.

TECH TIP

Backlinks are links back to your website or social media profiles. The more backlinks you have, the better. This is a large portion of how Google determines your relevance and your location in search engine results. You can build these backlinks yourself by commenting on other blogs or sharing via social media profiles.

NETWORKING IN THE DIGITAL AGE

Making connections and networking are becoming easier every day. Professional networking sites like LinkedIn give you the capability to easily connect with like-minded professionals and show your skills and ability to solve problems. Recruiters and hiring managers are increasingly using LinkedIn to find prime candidates to fill their roles. Demonstrating that you are knowledgeable about nursing topics and rising trends and issues in nursing can get you noticed and help advance your career.

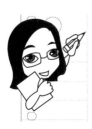

NERDY NOTE

Go to LinkedIn and try to connect with any former bosses or colleagues with whom you were on good terms when you left. Leave endorsements or recommendations on their profiles. Chances are high that they will do the same for you!

Many travel nurses use Twitter as a means of finding new work assignments. The world is their oyster, and they connect with new friends and eventual colleagues in an ever-growing social network built around 140 characters or less. If you are interested in having friends on a global scale and finding new and interesting opportunities in nursing, Twitter is where you want to be.

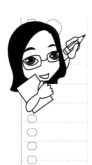

NERDY NOTE

To use Twitter to find travel nurse assignments, find and then follow nursing recruiters and job resources. Communicate with these account holders and let them know who you are and what you do. Pay attention to their tweets and reach out to them when you see an opportunity that you think you'd be great for. If you've established a good relationship with them, there's a good chance that they will contact you directly when they see an assignment you might be interested in.

Google+ continues to grow in popularity, with communities sprouting up everywhere. There are communities focusing on nursing in general or your preferred specialty. The integration with existing Google accounts and ever-growing array of Google web apps and tools makes this Google social networking site very appealing

Facebook has many pages and groups for nurses. Just remember that if you are going to use your personal Facebook page for networking with professionals, then you should probably make sure that your page's content is professional. It might be a good idea to create more than one profile so that you can connect with your family and friends on one account and your potential employers on another. But remember, on both accounts you should be mindful of the information you post. Once something is on the Internet, it's pretty much written in stone.

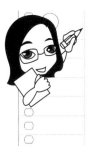

NERDY NOTE

A great Facebook group for travel nurses is called The Gypsy Nurse Caravan. Nurses can find fellow travel nurses to be their roommates, stop over on a long drive, or just grab a bite to eat. Nurses talk about what they like and dislike about assignments, their agencies, and the challenges they face on the road. It's a growing community of nurses who have each other's back.

ESTABLISHING YOUR NURSING BRAND

You're likely reading this heading and scratching your head a little bit. You're a nurse, not a product manufacturer. What the heck does "nursing brand" even mean, and how on earth do you establish it? It's understandable if you have this reaction. In the past, nurses have not had much difficulty in securing employment. Competition was not as heated when there weren't as many nursing schools and fewer trained and experienced nurses were on the scene. However, the days of getting a job just because you are a nurse are in the past in many areas, so it's important to establish a brand early so that you can set yourself apart from the crowd.

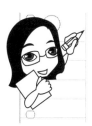

NERDY NOTE

Although there may be a statistical nursing shortage, many aren't feeling it. New grads and seasoned nurses alike are facing a tough job market in many areas. Having a nursing license no longer means that you'll always have a job.

"What exactly is a nursing brand?" you ask. Your nursing brand is your image, your motto, your mantra, your identity. It's what you stand for and your level of professionalism. It's your attitude and your goals. It's basically everything about you and your nursing career.

Your nursing brand is all that is awesome about you and what you wish to accomplish with your nursing career. You are the only one who can determine this, and it's up to you to establish it and make it so.

To be completely honest, I didn't think of having a nursing brand until after I started blogging. But nurses as individuals also have brands. You should think of yourself as an independent contractor, even if you work for a large health organization. You have to make yourself a marketable asset and resource so that a company sees value in you, whether you are content in your role or are seeking advancement.

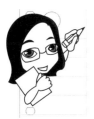

NERDY NOTE

Always be open to new opportunities. You never know when a great one is going to fall right in your lap. You need to be prepared to take advantage.

Even if you're gainfully and happily employed and love what you do right now, you still need to be aware of your personal brand as a professional nurse. Treat your career as a business and market yourself accordingly. Are you happy with your current income level, your current role, and your current opportunities for growth? Or do you want to do more in your nursing career? Do you want to grow in your profession? Do you want your business (your nursing career) to be a long-term success with constant growth, or do you want to stay exactly where you are now in your nursing career?

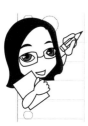

NERDY NOTE

These rules also totally apply if you are a nurse entrepreneur. Your brand could mean the difference between paying the bills or sleeping on someone else's couch. Establish your brand early and maintain it meticulously.

There is nothing wrong with being content in your current role as a nurse. If you are content with your current position, then you should pat yourself on the back. I'm envious of you—it would be so much easier to just be content. There would likely be a lot less stress in this world if we could all just be content. Then again, we'd also never innovate or seek improvements, and I'm pretty sure we'd all be sitting in the dark and trying to figure out fire, the wheel, and other silly things like that. Those crazy discontented ancestors of ours really stepped up to the plate on some of those things.

I sometimes wish that I could just be content. I sometimes wish that I could stop wanting to do a little bit more. I sometimes wish that I didn't care so much. Life would certainly be easier—but it would also be boring.

If you're like many other nurses, you can't just be content with the status quo. Your heart and head tell you that things could be better. You got into nursing because you wanted to make a difference, and you know that things could be done to improve the world around you.

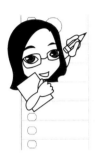

NERDY NOTE

You can expand your nursing horizons in ways other than climbing the health care career ladder. You may find that you are passionate about volunteering or writing. You define your own level of nursing success. Don't let anyone stand in the way of your career goals or tell you they aren't good enough, because you are the only person who knows what will make you happy.

For those of you who are not ready to settle or who want more out of life and your nursing career, personal branding is key to setting yourself apart from the rest of the nurses who are after the same success you are. You have to define yourself as a unique asset and market yourself as a vital piece of a health care organization's success. You have to believe in yourself and in the work you do now and can do in the future.

It's so important that you believe in yourself. If you don't believe in yourself, how on earth do you ever expect to convince anyone else to believe in you? The best tool nurses can have in their toolbox is confidence. Your patients, coworkers, and administration will value you for it. However, *do not confuse confidence with arrogance*, because no one will value you for that. You should be aware of your strengths and use them to provide the best patient care possible.

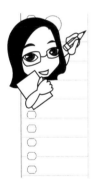

NERDY NOTE

As an assertive woman, I often believe that others confuse my confidence and assertiveness with arrogance. When I worked on the floor, this was an even bigger challenge. In my role in informatics, this quality is often seen as a huge asset. And although I still have to work to make sure I communicate appropriately and effectively, it's nice to have this trait seen as an asset rather than a character flaw. In my heart, I always knew that my assertiveness was a good thing, and it was one of the ways I was able to get into informatics.

Market yourself as a confident person. Even if you are not trying to get another job, use every professional encounter as an opportunity to show someone you're confident in the care you provide. Your confidence in your care will improve the relationships you have with your patients and coworkers, and you will be seen as a resource to others. You should always be aware of how others perceive you. You never know when an impression you've made can lead to bigger and better things for you and your career.

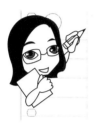

NERDY NOTE

Open lots of windows, because you never know when the door might close. If your current nursing role is eliminated or you can no longer perform it, you need to make sure that you are well prepared to move on and continue to support yourself by doing what you love.

Be yourself. This might mean being different. This might mean being bold. But be aware ahead of time that not everyone appreciates a confident nurse. Not everyone is confident in themselves, and their jealousy of your confidence will likely come out in a negative form or fashion. Because of this, there will always be naysayers. There will always be Debbie Downers. Be prepared for that.

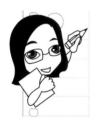

NERDY NOTE

Always carry an umbrella for protection against potential parade-rainers. My umbrella was social media. Your umbrella might be a favorite hobby or special place you like to go.

Actions speak louder than words. Rather than just dreaming up ideas, you need to dream them up and then put them into action. If you want to set yourself apart, you have to step out on the edge, be a little different, and shine a little brighter than all the other stars. As nurses, we already set ourselves apart from many people with the rigorous education we have attained, but you graduated with 100 other nurses who have the same credentials behind their names. Multiply that by some astronomical figure, and that's your competition.

I'll give you a great example of putting dreams into action. I wanted to work in nursing informatics. I built a blog, taught myself some basic database knowledge, and researched, researched, and researched. I did my BSN clinicals in an informatics setting and networked like crazy. Less than 3 months after I began seriously looking for an informatics role in nursing, I landed an awesome dream job where I am valued not only for my skills but for my opinions and insight. I get to be part of a great health care organization that is doing amazing things for the community, but I also get to be myself and pursue personal dreams and goals as well—all with my employer's full support.

Even if a blog isn't your cup of tea, you can still use technology to help establish your personal brand. Using LinkedIn can really help improve your brand. Take time to go to nursing groups and answer questions about topics that you know the answers to. If you don't know the answers, take the time to research them and share the information with the interested parties. Not only will you be increasing your nursing knowledge, but you will be establishing your credibility and your personal nursing brand with the online nursing community.

Determine what you want to accomplish in your nursing career and build your nursing brand around it. Branding is about what makes you unique. You have to show why your star shines a little brighter. Give your personal best and highlight what it is about *you* that is unforgettable, unmistakable, and irreplaceable as an employee. If you are interviewing for a job, you don't want the recruiters to put your resume in a pile. You want them to have conversations about you. You want them to see a spark in you that they didn't see in anyone else. You want them to call the other applicants and tell them to not even bother coming in.

DETERMINE YOUR VALUE AND SELL IT

You are probably sitting here confused at this point. Have you ever stopped and thought about what makes you unique, valuable, and an asset to a company? If you haven't, then now is the time. Make a list. Identify your top three personal attributes (examples include charisma, dedication, focus, teamwork, self-motivation, creativity, being a team player, leadership, and so on). Determine how these can be best applied to the nursing role you are after and work out your game plan. Write your nursing elevator pitch and be prepared to sell yourself whenever the chance arises.

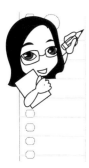

NERDY NOTE

An elevator pitch is a short monologue that you can spout off in about 30 seconds. Its name comes from the amount of time that you might spend with someone on an elevator. In this brief time frame, you should be able to give a good representation of who you are and what you stand for. Sometimes you only have a short period to make an impression, so always be prepared to tell people who you are and why you are awesome.

If you want others to see you as successful, you have to see yourself as successful first. Own your expertise today, and your dream job will likely find you in the near future!

ADAPTABILITY AND FLEXIBILITY IN THE WORKFORCE

Being able to quickly grasp new technologies is a fantastic job skill for any nurse. As a clinical informatics nurse, and just a nerdy nurse in general, I often find myself in situations where I'm being an evangelist for technology. I'll be spouting off about how fantastic some new innovation in software is or how much more efficient we are becoming when the nurses I am speaking with often just want me to fix their problem and move on so that they can stop dealing with the computer. Many of these nurses are talented and seasoned professionals who have no desire to use computers to improve the care their patients receive. In their opinion, they could get more done back in the days when they were able to jot down a few notes and actually spend time caring for the patients hands-on. These days they feel like they are caring more for the charts than they are the patients.

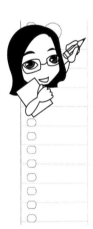

NERDY NOTE

Patients are sicker, computers are quicker, and technology isn't going anywhere.

You already know that technology is here to stay and that patients are getting sicker and sicker. In the back of your head, you know that computers are fast and you know what they can do. It's up to you to make computers work for you. Find ways to streamline your processes and use technology wherever it can improve your workflow.

Make it a personal goal to find one way each week that technology can save you time. Initially this change make take a little preparation, but in the long run you will have a lot more time to spend helping improve patient care.

I get it. I really do. Whenever I encounter these nurses, I smile, fix their problem, and try to take a few moments to show them how technology can make their job easier. If you're like most nurses, you just want to be able to take care of your patients without being weighed down by extra work. You want to be able to give your patients the attention they need, but at the same time, you know that you have to make compromises to ensure that you have adequate documentation.

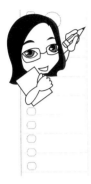

NERDY NOTE

If you ever feel like you are taking more care of the chart than the actual patient, then you may need to step back and reevaluate your workflow. I find that many nurses document way more than they actually need to and are often documenting things in more than one place. There is simply no need for this. If you documented on a patient's condition through an intervention note, there is no need to write another narrative nursing note. If you are doing this, stop—and add the extra minutes to other parts of your day.

MOVING BEYOND THE PAST

The words of nurses who believe that computers and electronic charts hinder their ability to do their job often echo in the back of my mind when I am thinking of ways to inspire others about why they should get excited about technology in health care. Perhaps nurses were able to get more done when they were using paper charts, but those same nurses will also admit that those patients were not nearly as sick. There were also not nearly the number of CMS regulations and Joint Commission on Accreditation of Healthcare Organizations (JCAHO) requirements to follow at the time either.

Yes, times were likely simpler when nurses documented their notes with pen and paper, but during those simpler days, we often were faced with the challenge of watching patients die of diseases that today we can cure. We also didn't wear gloves to protect ourselves from potentially deadly infections.

I hope you found this chapter motivating. You should now know some of the ways that technology can help you in your nursing career. Were you paying attention? Try to answer a few questions:

   ✛ What is personal branding, and why is it important for nurses?

   ✛ How can you use Twitter to enhance your resume?

   ✛ How can a grasp of technology make you a more desirable employee?

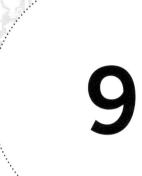

THE BIGGER PICTURE: TECHNOLOGY ISN'T GOING ANYWHERE

Many nurses are resistant to using technology and electronic medical records (EMRs), falling back on the tired excuse, "What happens when the system goes down?" Rather than focus on the benefits and positive aspects, they are quick to jump on the bandwagon of finding any flaw in the system and exploiting it. These naysayers are often frequent complainers about other topics as well and generally have a negative attitude. The problem isn't so much that they don't agree with the system or don't like it but that their attitude rubs off on others.

These nurses pollute the environments they work in and make others hesitant to move forward with adopting new technologies and digital change. They frown upon anyone who gets excited about learning something new and are often condescending and judgmental toward nurses who are training them to use new technologies.

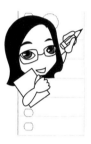

NERDY NOTE

Most nurses have worked with these types of people before. Some workplaces are free of them and are often therefore some of the best places to work. No one expects everyone to be a compliant robot, but there is a big difference between offering constructive criticism and just being negative.

The negative feelings and lashing out that they often exhibit are most often due to insecurity and fear. They fear the unknown. They fear what might happen if they can't adapt. They fear what might happen if the new change doesn't work, because they are comfortable with what they are currently doing. They lash out with anger and negativity rather than expressing their true concerns openly and honestly.

Their fear is understandable, but they should not let it take hold of them. They should have the self-confidence to learn whatever is necessary to take care of their patients. Many of these nurses are excellent at providing patient care, but their insecurities overwhelm them in other areas of the job.

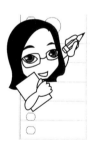

NERDY NOTE

If these nurses were focused on building their brands, they would be much less likely to feel overwhelmed. Other nurses in their midst can reduce their negative impact on the workplace by focusing on building their own brands and being positive and forward-thinking role models.

The best piece of advice that I can give nurses who react to change this way is that technology isn't going away. But at the same time, nurses aren't going anywhere either. Put your fear aside and replace it with an open mind and willingness to learn. Perception is reality, and you are completely in control of how you perceive things. Be aware of your perceptions and adapt them so that you react in a positive manner. This can help change your whole outlook on life and make you a happier person and a much better nurse.

But let's address the original concern that the naysaying nurse may have: "What if the system goes down?" If the system goes down, you will follow established downtime procedures. If the power goes out, backup generators will kick on, and the system will continue to run. What if the Zombie Apocalypse hits and all power and utilities cease to function? At that point, you've got bigger fish to fry than trying to chart on your patients. Initially you'll be manually bagging vented patients, and then you'll be fighting off turned patients with IV poles. You are a nurse; you can adapt. And in this situation, you had better adapt quickly, or all that nursing knowledge in your brain is going directly into the bellies of the walking dead.

CONGRATULATIONS! YOU'VE LEARNED A TON ABOUT TECHNOLOGY!

Let's get back to reality here for a moment and focus on those nurses who *do* want to change. If you saw technology as an inconvenient intimidation before picking up this book, I sincerely hope that your perception has changed. We've covered a lot of information about using technology and all that it can do to improve your life and the patient care you deliver. Let's take a few moments in this chapter to recap all we have learned.

We started out discussing all the information and resources that technology has to offer. Chapter 1 highlighted the reasons you should want the information, how patients can benefit from your skills with technology, and how you can use technology to obtain this information. We also touched on how technology can help you improve your nursing care, make you an asset to your employer, and allow you to be a resource to nurses and other staff. This chapter was all about learning how technology is a tool in your nursing arsenal and priming you to open your mind.

In Chapter 2, we talked about Google and the Internet. By now, you should know all about Google, both the search engine and the web apps the company owns. If you read this chapter and nothing else, you'd know ways that technology could improve your life. The ability to perform a well-executed Google search should be in every nurse's arsenal.

Chapter 3 was entirely devoted to social media and blogging. These are two areas that are very near and dear to my heart, so I hope it inspired you to get online and start a conversation. We talked about different social media platforms, including Twitter, Facebook, Google+, and LinkedIn. This chapter should have helped you learn that you can be discuss nursing-related issues and topics online with confidence as long as you are aware of HIPAA policies and maintain a professional tone.

If computers were intimidating to you before, hopefully they are less so after you read Chapter 4. We talked about computers and even a few tips and tricks that should save you some major time and frustration. You probably already own a computer, so we built upon this foundation. We also talked about some cool technology that we don't necessarily think of as being computers. If you don't want to go out and buy a Roku box or Apple TV right now, it's probably because you already went out and bought one while you were reading that chapter.

Chapter 5 should have you feeling way more confident about what you can do with a smartphone. We touched on a lot of areas, including how you can use a smartphone in nursing, great apps, different carriers, and operating systems. You've probably downloaded 100 apps since reading this chapter, and if you haven't, it's likely because you ran out of space on your phone and are ready for an upgrade.

Are you reading this book on a tablet? I hope that after reading Chapter 6, you really wish that you were. We talked about using tablets for nursing, their different features, and some tips and tricks to make tablet use a little more fun. By now you should have your tablet well accessorized and be a total advocate for tablet technology.

While you may have already been using EMRs and electronic documentation on a daily basis prior to reading this book, you may have not known the reasons for the push to adopt this technology. Hopefully you have a better appreciation for this technology after reading Chapter 7 and will look for ways that you can become more involved with your hospital's nursing informatics and education team to improve your interaction with EMRs. There are so many ways that EMRs can improve patient care, so I hope you're thinking about this movement a little more closely now.

As nurses, we should be very proud of what we do. We're professionals, and we do really great, vital work. I hope that Chapter 8's discussion of career advancement and professional pride helped give you ideas for ways to use technology to further your nursing career by using social media to enhance your resume, networking, establishing your nursing brand, and being adaptable in the workplace. Technology can help you advance to where you want to be in nursing or help maintain your current position if you are content in this role. Either way, use it to your benefit.

This final chapter focuses on encouraging you and other nurses to stop being dinosaurs. At the same time, I spend some time reassuring you that the well-seasoned nurse offers great value. I also tie everything together and focus on what's really important in nursing— advocating for patients, yourself, and your practice.

PATIENTS ARE SICKER AND COMPUTERS ARE QUICKER

Sometimes when I was working the night shift, coworkers would start talking about the "good old days" of paper charting. They'd describe how they could get their documentation done in just a few minutes and have so much time to care for their patients. They'd also describe the former (lower) levels of regulations and standards fondly. But during these reminiscing sessions, they'd forget to mention all the errors they may have made, all the improvements they've seen in their careers, and how much better we're able to paint a picture of the care we deliver.

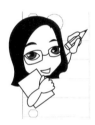

NERDY NOTE

We all know that nurses were responsible for far less back in the good old days and the patients weren't nearly as sick. We've come so far and are capable of so much more now. Why would we want to halt this progress? Let's keep the momentum going with technology.

The conversation would eventually turn to how much more "work" and responsibilities that nurses are tasked with these days. Not only are we responsible for significantly more charting than in the past, but we are doing so many more procedures and taking care of patients who are much sicker than they were in the past. People are living longer and are thus requiring more medical and nursing interventions during their hospital stays.

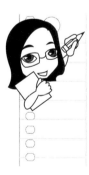

NERDY NOTE

Even though patients are sicker, they are spending less time in the hospital, and health care organizations are being reimbursed less and less. Everyone is being asked to do more with less, and nurses unfortunately have to bear the same burden. But with these increased responsibilities also come new technologies, such as the EMRs, smart pumps, and computerized inventories that we talked about earlier in the book. Use them to help you do your job and offset the heavy load when possible.

Technology allows nurses to be able to keep up with the ever-accelerating pace and automate some of the routine tasks we do. It also allows us to catalog information to better understand how we can care for patients. One of the greatest benefits of technology in direct patient care is the increased safety level. By having patients wear scannable bracelets that link to barcoded medications, we can ensure they are receiving only the medications intended for them.

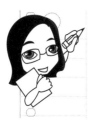

NERDY NOTE

Don't forget to educate your patients on the technologies you are using. Not only will they appreciate the time you took to explain this information, but they will also have increased confidence in the care you are providing.

Electronic charting gives nurses reminders to complete tasks that might otherwise be forgotten. I can remember when my hospital implemented hourly rounding documentation. It made many nurses get up and check on their patients much more often than they had before. Although most of the nurses thought they were doing a decent job before, this extra reminder of a needed task was enough to prompt them to make a round when they otherwise might not have. Most nurses may grumble about the additional fields to complete, but they understand the importance of checking on their patients and making sure that their needs are met.

TECH TIP

You're probably already making hourly rounds and documenting in a narrative note. Save yourself some time and document anything you might have made in a narrative note in your rounding interventions.

The intervention tracking capability of most EMR software has really come a long way. They often prompt the nurses and suggest tasks to them based upon their care plans. Instead of having to manually remember to key into different assessments, nurses add them as part of the patient's plan of care, and the nurses see a due date on the screen to remind them that these assessments should be completed.

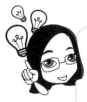

These reminders are great for pain medications. Many systems give you a reminder to check on the patient's pain level after administering pain medication. You can usually document on the patient's relief in an intervention with a few clicks rather than having to create a detailed nursing note.

With all the things that you have to do every day, it's impossible to keep everything straight in your head at any given time. It's important to understand that computers aren't meant to do your job for you, but they are meant to assist you. Computers can be a valuable resource if you recognize their benefits and take advantage of them. You should never forget that technology is a tool that clever nurses can use to help them deliver excellent patient care.

DON'T BE A DINOSAUR

Everyone knows why you don't have to fend off dinosaurs every day. But it's not like aliens came one day and took all the dinosaurs off the planet (unless you're talking with some of these ancient alien conspiracy folks). Dinosaurs died out due to a natural disaster. They're extinct because they couldn't adapt to their changing environment. Many of them were killed instantly by a possible meteor impact, but others held on a little longer and died more slowly and painfully of starvation.

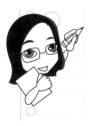

NERDY NOTE

Many well-seasoned nurses may feel like they are threatened with extinction. It's important that all nurses cement themselves as assets to their employers. I hope that this book has shared a few ways that technology can help you do this.

Technology can be a potential meteorite to a nursing career. If you don't adapt and learn how to maneuver technology in a new environment, then you too will "die off," while the nurses who adapt quickly replace you. But you know what happened to the dinosaurs who could adapt? They became birds. They evolved and changed over time and ultimately learned to spread their wings and fly.

Luckily for you, you're a bird, and you're learning to fly as you read these very words. Picking up this book is a step in the right direction toward making a positive change. By now you know all that technology can do for you. This is a big accomplishment in and of itself, but it's important that you don't stop now. Take charge in your own nursing career but also be an advocate to other nurses about the ways that technology can help them.

I've known several nurses in my day who have lost all passion. They do their nursing tasks and complete routines, but their hearts are no longer in the job. An informatics nursing friend of mine calls them "Appliance Nurses"—nurses who are only working so they can afford their next major appliance. It's unfortunate, but these dinosaurs stomp around and take up space, warm chairs, and refuse to give more than the bare minimum. They have no interest in learning anything new and often discourage others from furthering their education.

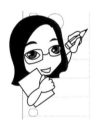

NERDY NOTE

Even a good nurse can be a dinosaur. Saying, "I've been here forever and things will never change" is a cop-out. Never underestimate the power of a nurse determined to change things.

THERE IS NO CONSPIRACY TO PUNISH THE WELL-SEASONED NURSE

One of the biggest arguments I hear against embracing EMRs and other nursing-related technology is that it's an attempt to push well-seasoned nurses out the door. In reality, this couldn't be further from the truth. An EMR is meant to enhance patient care, not punish you for wanting to provide it. Each nurse offers different experiences, perspectives, and knowledge levels to help the health care process flow. Young nurses may be more experienced with computers, but watching them try to put in a Foley catheter is like a bad comedy movie—it's not funny; it's not useful; it's just frustrating. Team up with those nurses and show them the tips and tricks you've learned in your years of experience at the bedside (and what you've learned from this book!), and they will be happy to help you master the computer.

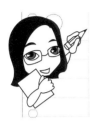

NERDY NOTE
Experienced nurses should speak up and offer their help during EMR implementation. Your expertise can be utilized to create better nursing documentation.

Many nurses find it difficult to accept change and move past "the way it's always been." EMRs are a huge adaptation for anyone to make, and if you're already set in your ways and are resistant to change, you are just going to make your life more difficult. Seasoned nurses may feel like they are being targeted because their skill sets are not as technologically strong. However, they are just as capable of becoming experts on the new systems as any other nurses.

Those young whippersnapper hotshots on the computer need the help of nurses who have spent time in the trenches. Nursing is a team effort. Seasoned nurses should lend their expertise when needed and be prepared to absorb new knowledge daily. It has been said before that a nurse who knows everything is a very dangerous nurse. Use every day to learn something new. Some days, that new thing should involve technology!

BE AN ADVOCATE FOR YOUR PATIENTS, YOUR PROFESSION, AND YOUR PRACTICE

Nursing is a difficult job that is constantly changing and forcing us to adapt to deliver the best care for the patients we serve. It is not enough that we carry out orders and complete documentation. We must make sure that we are putting patients' best interests first and advocating for their wants and needs.

Technology can give you an advantage in your personal and professional life and can help you better meet the needs of your patients. We must not forget the reasons we got into nursing or let the distractions of change cause us to become jaded and bitter. Patients suffer when nurses struggle to cope with evolving digital change. We lose good nurses due to lack of support and lack of understanding of the difficulty associated with such changes.

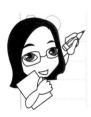

NERDY NOTE
Don't forget, technology can be a whole lot of fun too! Nursing is hard work, and sometimes it's nice to relax and just play around with technology.

In the beginning, embracing new technologies can be overwhelming and far from easy, but with time you will find that after making the initial adjustments and opening your mind to learning, the next new steps will come much easier. Do not hesitate to ask your peers questions. Never underestimate the power of a well-executed Google search. And never pass up an opportunity to learn a new skill or to use a new technology.

If there is one constant in nursing and health care, it is that there will always be change. Adaptability is one of the single most important traits of a successful nurse. This profession has no room for people who are "set in their ways." Providing good nursing care sometimes requires making small sacrifices.

You should be very proud of yourself right now for making the effort to learn more about technology. Just by reading this book, you've already learned so much and now have the tools to learn even more. We've had nine information-packed chapters, and you made it to the very end! But don't stop here, because technology is constantly changing and evolving. Make it a part of your life and use it to improve the care you deliver. Be an advocate for technology to other nurses and help your patients cope with evolving digital change.

I hope you've learned that technology is meant to make your life easier and can help you be a better nurse if you let it. This was a fantastic journey, and I'm so happy you came along. Thank you, from the bottom of my heart, for taking the time to read this book and to learn a little more about technology.

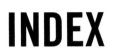

INDEX

W

X–Y–Z

U–V

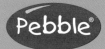

Our Community Helpers

Construction Workers Help

by Tami Deedrick

Consulting Editor: Gail Saunders-Smith, PhD

CAPSTONE PRESS
a capstone imprint

Pebble Books are published by Capstone Press,
1710 Roe Crest Drive, North Mankato, Minnesota 56003
www.capstonepub.com

Library of Congress Cataloging-in-Publication Data
Cataloging-in-Publication information is on file with the Library of Congress.
ISBN 978-1-4765-3950-8 (library binding)
ISBN 978-1-4765-5154-8 (paperback)
ISBN 978-1-4765-6011-3 (ebook PDF)

Note to Parents and Teachers

The Our Community Helpers set supports national social studies
standards for how groups and institutions work to meet individual
needs. This book describes and illustrates construction workers.
The images support early readers in understanding the text. The
repetition of words and phrases helps early readers learn new
words. This book also introduces early readers to subject-specific
vocabulary words, which are defined in the Glossary section. Early
readers may need assistance to read some words and to use the
Table of Contents, Glossary, Read More, Internet Sites, and Index
sections of the book.

Printed in the United States of America in North Mankato, Minnesota.
112018   001159

Table of Contents

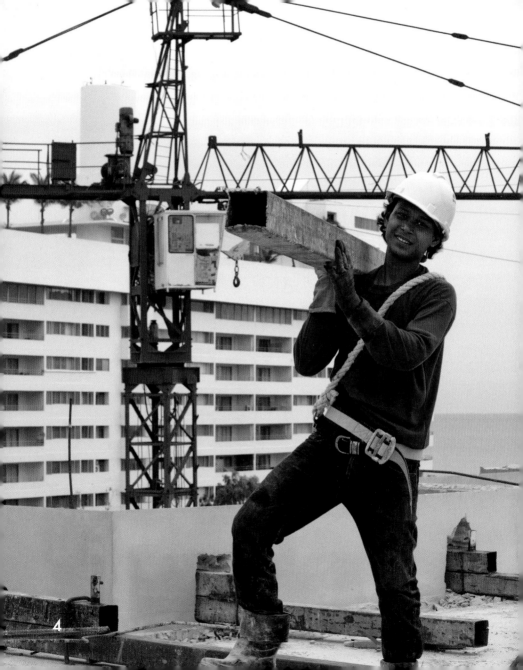

What Is a Construction Worker?

Construction workers are people who build things. They build homes, schools, and skyscrapers. They also build roads and bridges.

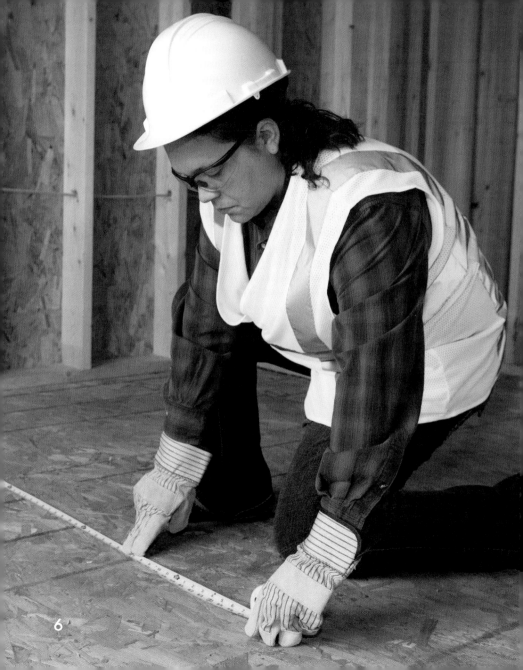

What Construction Workers Do

Construction workers dig, pound, cut, and measure. They follow plans drawn by architects or engineers.

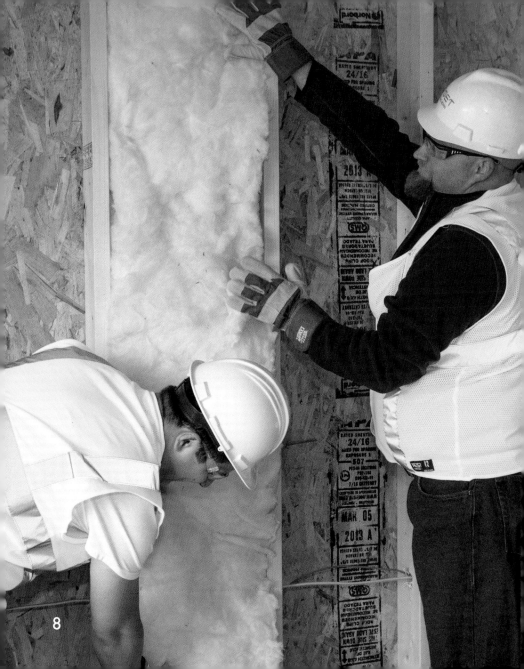

Construction workers work on job sites. They work together in crews. Everyone has a job to do. Framers build walls. Roofers nail shingles to roofs.

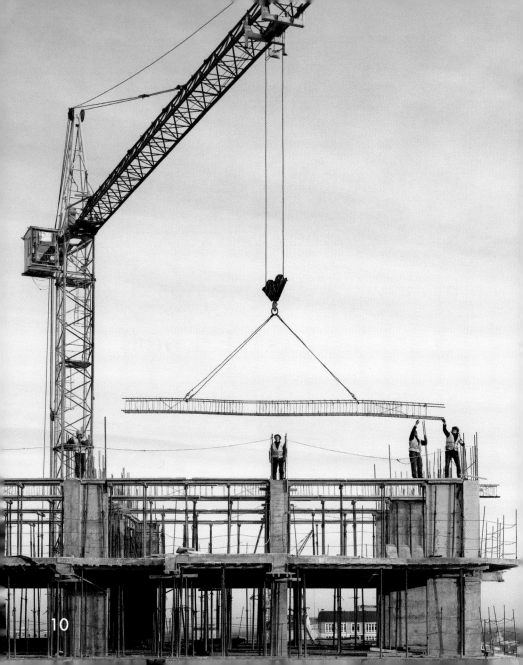

Construction workers use big machines. They drive bulldozers to move dirt. Cranes lift heavy supplies to high places.

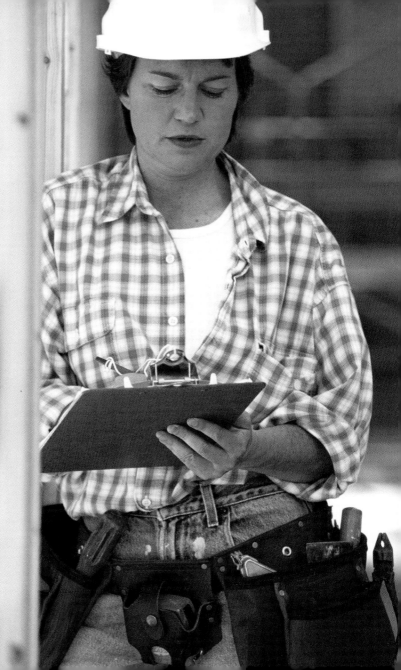

Clothes and Tools

Construction workers use many tools. They use saws to cut and shovels to dig. A tool belt holds a hammer, nails, and tape measure.

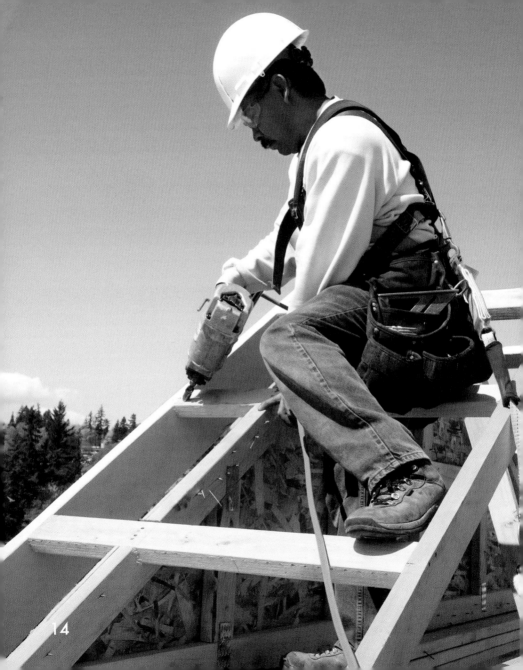

Construction workers wear special clothing to keep them safe. Hard hats protect their heads from falling objects.

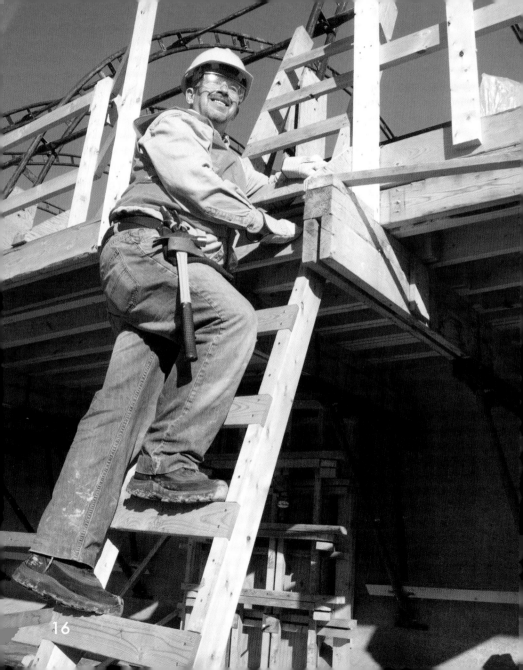

Other clothing is important too. Safety glasses keep dirt and debris out of eyes. Thick gloves and heavy boots protect hands and feet.

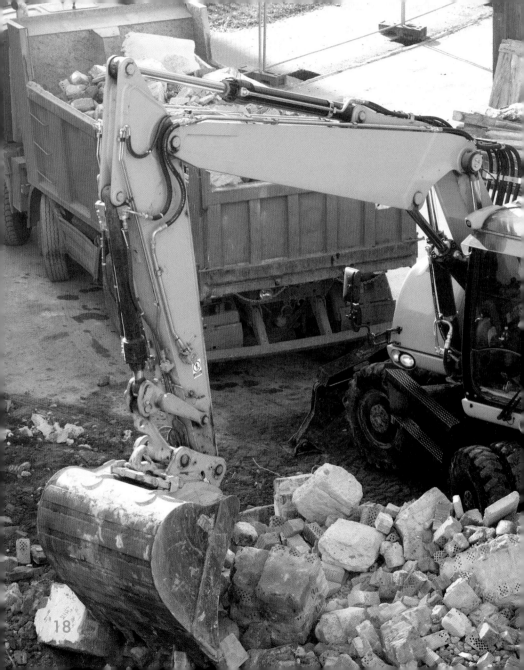

Taking Things Down

Some construction crews
take down old buildings.
Workers smash walls with
a wrecking ball. Excavators
take away huge pieces.

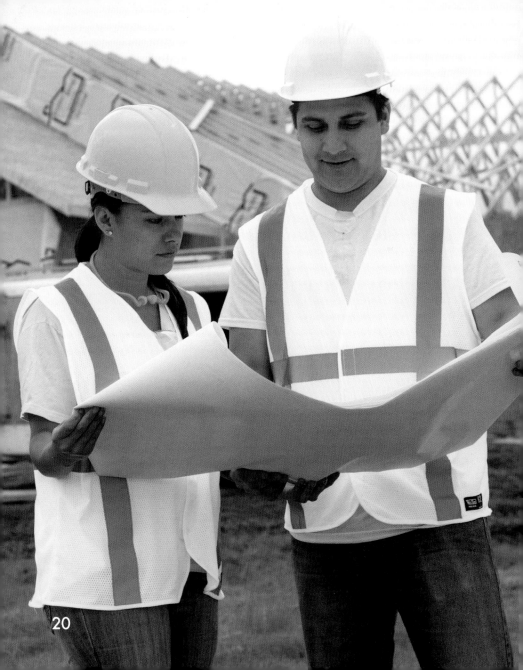

Construction Workers Help

Construction workers build new buildings and roads. Construction workers help communities grow.

Glossary

architect—a person who designs and draws plans for buildings, bridges, and other construction projects

community—a group of people who live in the same area

debris—the scattered pieces of something that has been broken or destroyed

engineer—a person who uses science and math to plan, design, or build

excavator—a machine used to dig in the earth

skyscraper—a very tall building made of steel, concrete, and glass

Read More

Heos, Bridget. *Let's Meet a Construction Worker.* Community Helpers. Minneapolis: Millbrook Press, 2013.

McGill, Jordan. *Buildings.* Community Helpers. New York: AV2 by Weigl, 2012.

Troupe, Thomas Kingsley. *Knock It Down!* Destruction. North Mankato, Minn.: Capstone Press, 2014.

Internet Sites

FactHound offers a safe, fun way to find Internet sites related to this book. All of the sites on FactHound have been researched by our staff.

Here's all you do:

Visit *www.facthound.com*

Type in this code: 9781476539508

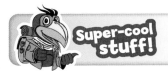

Check out projects, games and lots more at
www.capstonekids.com

Index

Word Count: 171
Grade: 1
Early-Intervention Level: 20

Editorial Credits
Erika L. Shores, editor; Gene Bentdahl, designer; Charmaine Whitman,
production specialist

Photo Credits
Capstone Studio: Karon Dubke, cover, 6, 8, 20; Dreamstime: Chaloemkiad, 4,
Dpproductions, 14; Glow Images: Flirt/Corbis/Curtis/Strauss, 12;
Shutterstock: ivvv1975, 10, Jaroslaw2313, 16, JMiks, 18